EMPTY CRIBS

THE IMPACT OF SMOKING ON CHILD HEALTH

Michael Dean

First Edition

Arts and Sciences Publishing
Frederick

EMPTY CRIBS

THE IMPACT OF SMOKING ON CHILD HEALTH

Arts and Sciences Publishing
5257 Buckeystown Pike, #173
Frederick, MD 21704 U.S.A.

orders@artsciencepub.com
http://www.artsciencepub.com

Library of Congress Control Number: 2006906824

ISBN-10 0-9786907-0-2
ISBN-13 978-0-9786907-0-0

First edition 2006
Printed in the United States of America

Dean, Michael
Empty Cribs-The impact of smoking on child health
Includes bibliographic references and index.

Praise for Empty Cribs

"This well researched, very readable book can save lives. If someone you love smokes and is planning to become a parent, make them a present of this book, but not before you read it yourself and get angry at how much more could be done by governments to prevent the leading single cause of death in our time."
Professor Simon Chapman, Editor Tobacco Control

"You knew tobacco smoke hurt children, but you probably never knew how much. Now you do."
Joe Cherner, founder of BREATHE-- Bar and Restaurant Employees Advocating Together for a Healthy Environment.

"Dr. Michael Dean has put the spotlight on an often overlooked aspect of the tragedy of cigarette smoking: the devastating effects it can have on children. By raising awareness of the causal relationship between exposure to cigarette smoke and infant mortality—including Sudden Infant Death Syndrome (SIDS) this book performs and important service. Parents and prospective parents need the information in this book. By eliminating exposure to cigarette smoke, nearly hundreds if not thousands deaths from SIDS alone could be prevented annually in the United States. Adding in the deaths from low birth weight, lung infections and asthma, Dr. Dean estimates that annually there are over 4,000 smoking-related preventable infant deaths each year. The take home message: cigarette smoke can kill your children."
Dr. Elizabeth Whelan
President, American Council on Science and Health

Contents

Introduction

Michael was roused out of his dream by the sun streaming into his face. The mockingbird outside was chattering up a storm. It seemed like weeks since he had slept this soundly. It had been weeks! Six weeks and two days, to be exact, since his daughter was born. The baby slept through the night! Suddenly that thought disturbed him. Was the baby all right? He rolled out of bed and walked down the hall to the nursery with increasing agitation.

His wife awoke to a penetrating cry of anguish…

Every day, in the United States, an average of seven babies die of sudden infant death syndrome (SIDS). These tragedies destroy familes and account for an enormous amount of heartache. What if there was a way to prevent this awful fate from happening to these families? What if the lives of other infants who die in the womb, in the maternity ward, and in homes could be saved? There is! **Maternal smoking and exposure of baby and mother to secondhand smoke is the most common preventable cause of infant mortality.**

In 1938, publicity surrounding the deaths of children working in factories led to public support of changes in the working conditions of children. The public outcry led to the passage of Federal child labor laws and to a vast improvement in children's education and quality of life. Today thousands of unborn children in the womb and after birth are exposed to poisons from tobacco smoke. Smoking contributes to the death of four thousand infants each year in the United States, including a large portion of the babies that die of SIDS. In addition, most people who acquire a long-term or life-long addiction to tobacco begin smoking as children.

Adults know that a pregnant woman should not smoke and that babies should not be exposed to smoke. However, the problem has been poorly addressed. Better education of parents is needed and action should be taken to help women quit smoking before they become pregnant. For those who feel this is an important issue, is it enough to quit smoking, pay your taxes, and warn your children not to smoke?

This book presents information on the effects of smoking on the health of children and mothers, and offers solutions to reduce infant mortality. *Empty Cribs* exposes a tragic situation and provides practical solutions to improve health. Economic choices are offered (which we can all use) to encourage companies and states to do a better job at preventing childhood tobacco use, maternal smoking, and infant mortality. Smoking in the workplace has been banned in several states and for the first time in thirty years, the number of deaths from cancer has declined. Through individual action exposure of children to smoke can be reduced, lessening the tragedy of infant mortality in our country.

Young cigar makers in Engelhardt & Co. Three boys looked under 14. Labor leaders told me in busy times many small boys and girls were employed. Youngsters all smoke. Tampa, Fla. 01/27/1909

Photograph 1909- Lewis W. Hine. Unedited caption by L.W. Hine.

Hine was one of America's pre-eminent early photographers. His series of photographs showing the consequences of child labor had enormous impact on public opinion.

Source: National Archives.

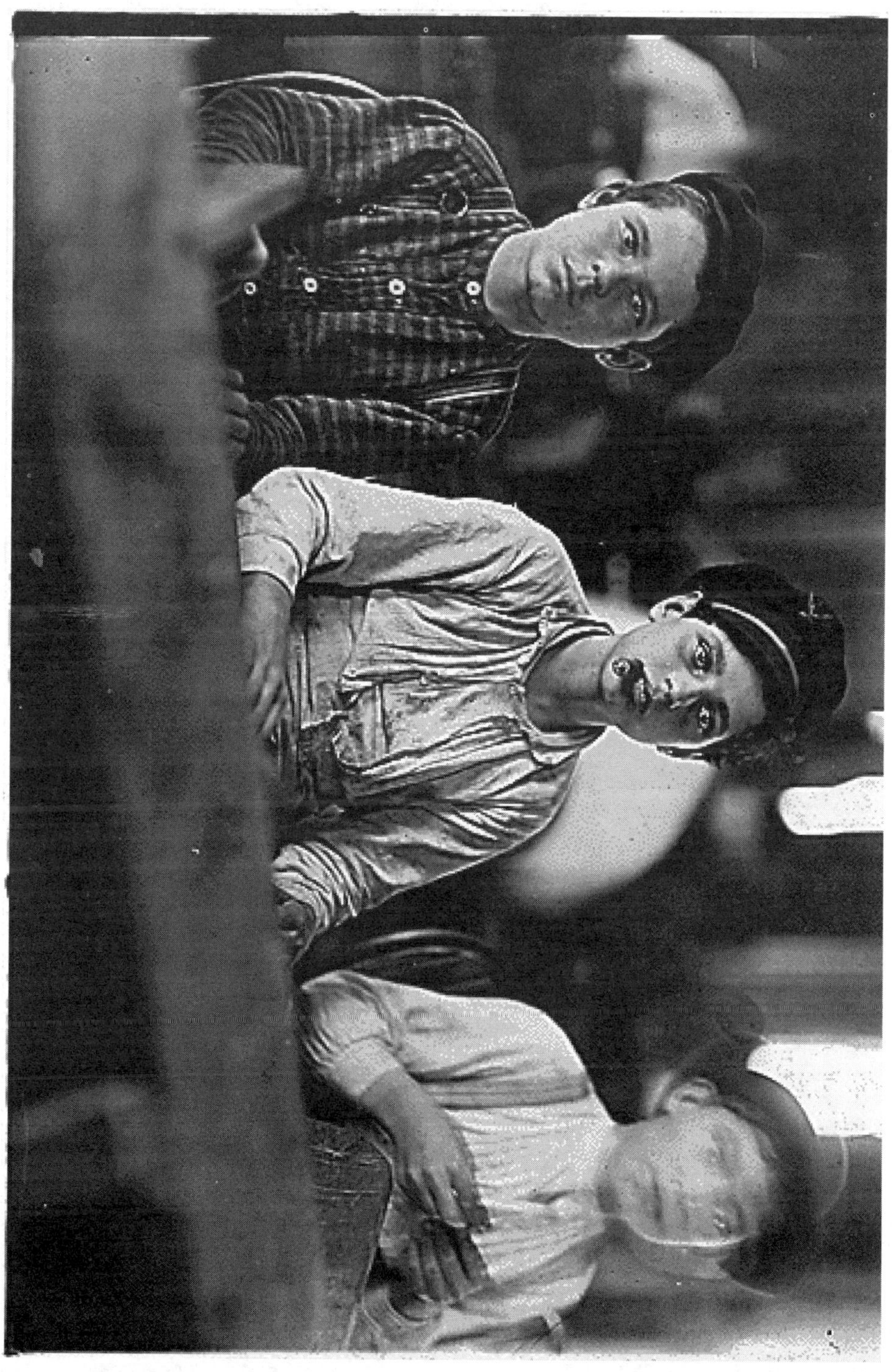

Chapter 1. Tobacco and Children

"If they have lips, we want them"

"At the outset it should be said that we are presently, and I believe unfairly, constrained from directly promoting cigarettes to the youth market ... [I]f our company is to survive and prosper, over the long term we must get our share of the youth market...Thus[,] we need new brands designed to be particularly attractive to the young smoker, while ideally at the same time appealing to all smokers[.] ... Perhaps these questions may be best approached by consideration of factors influencing pre-smokers to try smoking, learn to smoke and become confirmed smokers."

Claude Teague, Assistant Chief in R&D at R.J. Reynolds "Some Thoughts About New Brands of Cigarettes for the Youth Market," 1973.

The tobacco companies have always known that the young smoker is essential to their business. Get them to smoke your brand early and they will often stick with it. These companies have carefully researched smoking in children as young as five years old. One executive, when asked what age should be targeted, said, "If they have lips, we want them." One of the large Canadian tobacco businesses, the Imperial Tobacco Company, set out to learn what makes young people smoke. Their effort, called "Project 16" assembled focus groups of smoking preteen and adolescent boys and girls to better understand this market group.

In 2006, about three million adolescents will smoke almost a billion packs of cigarettes. Over one million children begin smoking each year at an average age of fourteen-and-a-half and 86 percent of them will smoke one of the three most heavily advertised brands. Access to tobacco by minors, although illegal, is not a problem. Children get cigarettes at home and from friends, and despite current laws, kids routinely buy them in stores.

A recent survey by students in Oldham County, Michigan, found six hundred tobacco ads in stores in their small town - part of the $15 billion spent each year to attract new smokers. Children are regularly exposed to tobacco ads. Cigarettes and smokeless tobacco are advertised in many magazines and are on display in grocery and convenience stores and at entertainment events. Very detailed research goes into these marketing campaigns. Tobacco use is widely shown in movies - even in films rated PG and PG-13. Lawmakers have largely driven ads out of magazines expressly written for children and have gotten rid of smoking cartoon characters. What is lacking is a concerted consumer effort to cut down on tobacco marketing and to change the policies of companies that advertise and sell tobacco products.

Children and Nicotine Addiction

Considerable effort has gone into understanding why kids start to smoke. Children ages ten to seventeen want to appear grown-

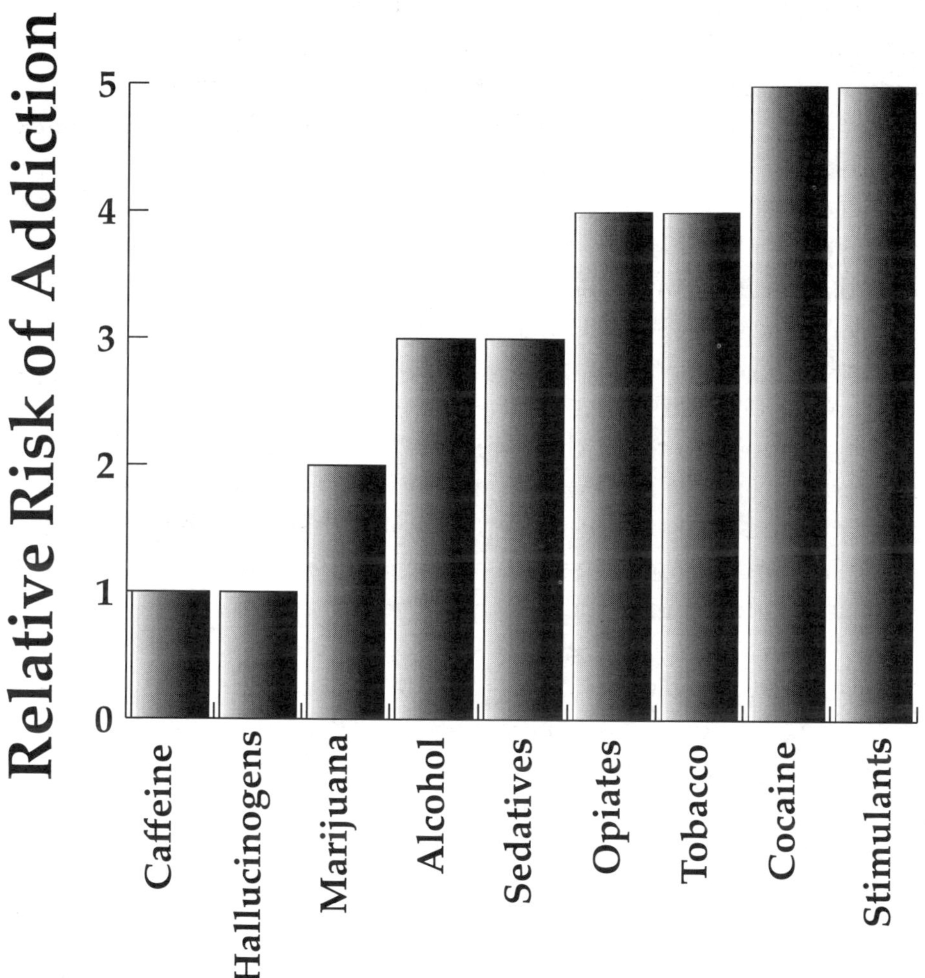

Figure 1.1 Ranking of commonly used drugs according to a scale of potential for addiction known as the relative risk of addiction: 1 represents the lowest risk and 5, the highest. Tobacco/nicotine has been given a score of 4.

up and are intensely curious about the things that adults do. They see adults smoking in their homes, in public and in movies. When they can, children get their hands on magazines that young men, women and adults read, such as *Cosmopolitan, Maxim* and *Playboy*. There, they see attractive models smoking. Of course, they also see tobacco ads in *Time, Newsweek, Sports Illustrated, People* and virtually all fashion magazines. Some magazines with cigarette ads can be found even in our middle schools and high schools. Virtually every convenience store, grocery store and gas station displays tobacco products, giving young people the impression that smoking is a normal part of adult life.

Schools do teach our children that smoking is addictive and causes cancer. But most children think they can try a few and quit anytime, and they are not concerned with what might happen to them in the distant future. Cigarettes are cheap, available and forbidden, so many children give them a try.

But why have cigarettes achieved such a foothold on the young? Why do so many young people become addicted? Cigarettes deliver a small dose of the addictive drug nicotine, which stimulates specialized cells in the brain. This causes the hormone adrenaline to be released, increasing the heart rate, and making the smoker alert. The smoker feels a mild euphoria, especially with the first few doses. Nicotine also stimulates the 'reward pathway' of the brain, creating a pleasurable sensation. Heroin, cocaine and marijuana also stimulate the reward pathway. The effects of nicotine wear off in an hour or two, and larger or more frequent doses are needed to get the same effect. Once the brain has adapted to nicotine, the smoker is dependant, or addicted.

Nicotine is addictive physically and psychologically, just like heroin and cocaine. Nicotine does not produce an intense high like these other drugs. But a smoker will continue to smoke even after he or she wants to quit, and smokers will often continue despite their doctor's advice - or even following heart attacks or lung cancer treatment. The majority of smokers want to quit and most have tried

Evidence that a Drug is Addictive

- **The drug binds to specific nerve cells in the brain**. Nicotine is in fact one of the best-studied of the drugs affecting the brain. It simulates the signaling of specific nerve cells.

- **There are physical withdrawal symptoms**. Most smokers, after they stop using nicotine, experience physical symptoms, including nervousness, headaches, decreased heart rate, and insomnia.

- **Users fail to quit despite real health risks.** Nicotine addicts continue their habit despite its obvious effect on their life, even when told that they will likely die as a consequence.

many times. Addiction researchers have attempted to rank drugs according to a scale known as the "relative risk of addiction." The relative risk of addiction for nicotine is as high as that for opiates like heroin and almost as high as for cocaine and other stimulants.

Nicotine replacement therapy is the most common method for treating cigarette addiction. Nicotine patches, gums and nasal sprays are effective because they replace the craving for the drug. This allows the individual to try to break the habit of smoking. Once that is accomplished the person can gradually cut out the nicotine to complete the process. However, habits acquired at a young age and practiced for years are hard to break. Approximately 20 to 30 percent of individuals quit smoking for at least six months following nicotine replacement therapy. Enrolling in a counseling program increases the likelihood of quitting successfully. Recently, antianxiety drugs such as bupropion (the generic name for Zyban and Wellbutrin) have been found to be effective in helping people quit smoking. And using an antianxiety drug and nicotine replacement together is even more effective than either therapy alone.

Health care providers routinely observe a great deal of difference in the success of people trying to stop smoking. Some people can give up cigarettes quite readily, while others try to quit and fail many times. Scientific studies, particularly studies of twins, show that part of the difference in the degree of nicotine addiction is genetic. In other words, some individuals are more likely than others to become addicted to nicotine and to stay hooked. Part of this difference involves the length of time that the drug remains in the body. Some peoples' bodies remove nicotine from the blood very rapidly, whereas others do so more slowly.

The severity of a person's nicotine addiction can be assessed by a simple questionnaire, developed by Dr. Karl Fagerstrom. The test is called the Fagerstrom Test for Nicotine Dependence. People who smoke their first cigarette within thirty minutes of waking up and smoke over twenty cigarettes per day usually score as "highly addicted" on this test. The test can be useful in guiding an individual smoking cessation plan. Fewer smokers succeed in quitting 'cold turkey,' and many of these smokers may require more intensive therapy or may require several attempts before they stop smoking.

Fagerstrom Test for Nicotine Dependence

______1. How soon after you awake do you smoke your first cigarette?

0. After 30 minutes
1. Within 30 minutes

______2. Do you find it difficult to refrain from smoking in places where it is forbidden, such as the library, theater, or doctor's office?

0. No
1. Yes

______3. Which of all the cigarettes you smoke in a day is the most satisfying?

0. Any other than the first one in the morning
1. The first one in the morning

______4. How many cigarettes a day do you smoke?

0. 1-15
1. 16-25
2. More than 26

______5. Do you smoke more during the morning than during the rest of the day?

0. No
1. Yes

______6. Do you smoke when you are so ill that you are in bed most of the day?

0. No
1. Yes

______7. Does the brand you smoke have a low, medium, or high nicotine content?

0. Low
1. Medium
2. High

______8. How often do you inhale the smoke from your cigarette?

0. Never
1. Sometimes
2. Always

SCORING INSTRUCTIONS: Add up your responses to all the items. Total scores should range from zero to eleven, where seven or greater suggests physical dependence on nicotine.

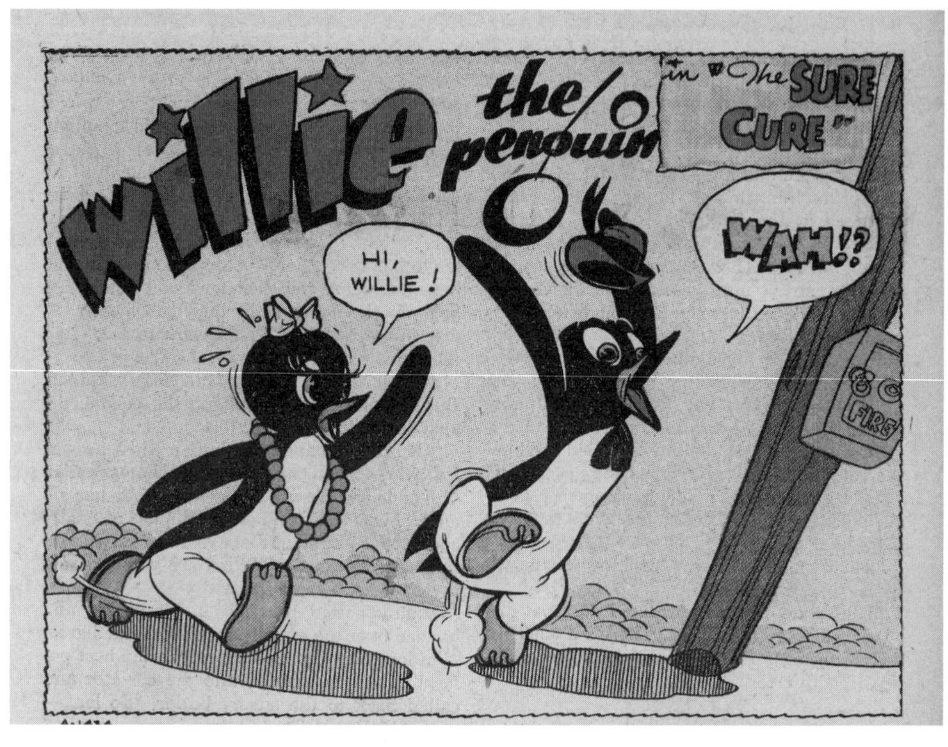

Figure 1.2 Willie the KOOL penguin comic from 1951. Featuring the Kool cigarette mascot.

Smoking rates among underage people have declined significantly in the last few years. In 1995, 35 percent of high school students were smokers, a number that declined to 22 percent in 2003, the last date that data is available from the Centers for Disease Control (CDC). A separate study indicates that the decrease has flattened out in the last two to three years. Disturbingly, the rate of smoking of eighth grade students, seen as the bellwether for future smokers, has remained constant. Experts attribute the continued high rate of smoking among ten- to fourteen- year-old children to a reduction in spending by the states on smoking education programs and an increase in tobacco marketing from $6.7 billion in 1998 to $15 billion in 2003.

Among fourteen- to eighteen-year-olds, white females have the highest rates of smoking, at 27 percent. Minorities smoke less, with 11 percent of African American female high school students smoking, and 19 percent of African American males and 18 percent of Hispanics. However, smoking rates differ dramatically by both educational background and economic status. Of women with sixteen or more years of education who gave birth in 2002, only 2 percent smoke, but 25 percent of those with less than eleven years of education smoked during their pregnancy. An amazing 43 percent of undereducated white women smoke during pregnancy. People with incomes below the poverty level also have significantly higher rates of smoking.

The government and private foundations are educating young people about the dangers of smoking and are helping people to quit. Every state has laws restricting smoking and tobacco sales, and tobacco products are heavily taxed. Lawsuits against tobacco companies have resulted in the payment of billions of dollars for the damages caused by cigarettes. Despite all this effort, tobacco advertising is still pervasive, access to cigarettes is easy and the rate of smoking in young people has remained high. Experts believe further reductions can be achieved by continuing to air anti-smoking ads, by raising the price of cigarettes, by restricting smoking in films to R-rated movies, by eliminating tobacco use in the workplace - and especially in bars, restaurants and music clubs - and by enforcing restrictions on tobacco sales to minors. However, the influence of family and community on children's choices is very strong. In households and families where there are no smokers, the children are far less likely to smoke.

Chapter 2. Smoking and Infant Mortality

The Unspoken Toll of Tobacco on Children

In 1994 Drs. C. Andrew Aligne and Jeffrey J. Stoddard published an important study in *The Archives of Pediatric and Adolescent Medicine* entitled "*Tobacco and Children.*" The article estimated the number of children who die from illnesses caused in part by exposure to tobacco. According to their calculations an astonishing 6400 children under eighteen die from the effects of their parents' smoking. This fact makes tobacco the number one preventable cause of death - greater than accidents, drowning, fires, choking, and poisoning combined.

The effects of smoking on children begin from the time they are conceived. If the mother smokes or breathes in smoke, the nicotine, carbon monoxide and other toxins present in the smoke reach the developing child. Maternal smoking dramatically affects development of the fetus and results in lower birth weight. This effect has been demonstrated by numerous scientific studies conducted since 1957. The tobacco industry, always trying to put a positive spin on things, tried to convince women that lower birth weight was an advantage and would make delivery easier! Unfortunately, low birth weight is a major risk factor for serious infant conditions such as respiratory problems and premature death.

One of the best-studied connections between smoking and childhood mortality involves SIDS. In 1992, the United States Environmental Protection Agency (EPA) found a link between secondhand smoke and SIDS. The California EPA conducted an extensive study of smoking and SIDS and found that both maternal smoking and exposure of babies to smoking were risk factors for SIDS. In 1997, the California study estimated that smoking caused between 1900 and 2700 SIDS deaths in the United States. Ever since the 1992 EPA study, the tobacco industry has sought to discredit the link between smoking and SIDS. However, in 2006, the United States Surgeon General released a report, "The Health Consequences of Involuntary Exposure to Tobacco Smoke." This report leaves no doubt:

> **Children exposed to secondhand smoke are at an increased risk for sudden infant death syndrome (SIDS), acute respiratory infections, ear problems, and more severe asthma. Smoking by parents causes respiratory symptoms and slows lung growth in their children.**

Despite the fact that over 2500 children die of SIDS in the United States each year, SIDS is a poorly understood and complicated disorder influenced by genetics and the environment. Campaigns to change the sleeping habits of babies, particularly advising parents to place babies on their back on a firm mattress, have led to dramatic reductions in SIDS cases in the United States and Europe.

Sweden implemented a SIDS education and prevention program, and they have one of the lowest rates of infant mortality in the world. A 2004 study looked at the remaining SIDS deaths occurring in Sweden since the program was started. The research found that babies exposed to smoke now have a four times greater risk for SIDS. The percentage of SIDS victims whose mothers smoked rose to 68 percent in a country where only 19 percent of the population smokes. So, with the reduced number of children sleeping on their stomachs, the most dangerous preventable risk factor for SIDS is now smoking! Similar studies conducted in Colorado and North Carolina also found a significant association between SIDS and smoking. These studies also found that, like in Sweden, efforts to reduce SIDS have been effective because the sleep position recommendations are being followed. However, the proportion of deaths due to smoking has increased. Health experts have published studies in top medical journals estimating that as many as 60 percent of SIDS cases, approximately two thousand deaths in the United States, can be prevented if we protect unborn children and babies from tobacco and nicotine exposure.

While the most serious adverse effects on health are seen in babies born to smoking mothers, secondhand smoke exposure also causes childhood disease. Fathers who smoke pose significant threats to their children, increasing the risk of SIDS and birth complications. Children sleeping in bed with their parents have been shown to be at risk for SIDS. But some studies show that this is true only when the child sleeps with a parent who smokes. One study by the European Concerted Action on SIDS found that babies who sleep with smoking mothers have an eighteen times greater risk of SIDS. Therefore, a child should never sleep in a room with a smoker.

Stoddard and Aligne's results updated

Drs. Aligne and Stoddard used data from 1980 to 1989 to make their estimates of the number of children who die from tobacco. They documented five principal causes of death due to smoking; SIDS, complications of low birth weight, household fires, asthma, and respiratory infections. Updated numbers and estimates indicate that a figure of four thousand deaths per year is currently more accurate.

SIDS. As discussed above, smoking by the mother and exposure of the infant to secondhand smoke are major risk factors for SIDS. Aligne and Stoddard estimated that smoking caused 36 percent of the 5500 SIDS deaths in 1989. By the year 2000, the rate of SIDS had dropped dramatically to 2543 deaths per year, due to efforts to educate parents on sleeping position from the *Back to Sleep* campaigns. Also, the percentage of mothers who smoke has declined from the 28 percent figure Aligne and Stoddard used, to between 12 to 20 percent today. The reduction in smoking mothers also contributed to the decline in SIDS. From a 2005 study of SIDS in Colorado for the years 1989 to 1998, it can be estimated that 23 percent of SIDS cases are attributed to smoking exposure. Using the more conservative 23 percent figure provides an estimate of 585 SIDS deaths per year in the United States attributed to smoking.

Low birth weight. A mother who smokes has a much higher chance of having a baby born with a low birth weight. Such babies are more likely to suffer from a number of health problems and have a higher incidence of death. In 2002, 314,077 babies were born weighing less than 2500 grams (5.5 pounds), meeting the definition of low birth weight. The mortality rate for these children is fifty-five deaths for every thousand babies in European American children and seventy eight deaths per thousand African Americans babies. Using the lower fifty-five out of one thousand number and the estimate that maternal smoking is responsible for 18 percent of low birth weight infants gives 3109 deaths per year caused by smoking.

Fires. About half of all household fires resulting in childhood deaths are caused by smoking. Aligne and Stoddard estimated that smoking causes 130 fatal childhood fire deaths and kids playing with cigarette lighters causes another 120 deaths. These numbers have remained virtually unchanged in the last ten years.

Asthma. Exposure to secondhand smoke is harmful to all infants and children with respiratory problems. The most common childhood lung disease is asthma. Childhood asthma deaths have increased in the United States to 223 per year. Approximately 14 percent of childhood asthma deaths are caused by smoking, according to Aligne and Stoddard, yielding thirty-one fatalities.

Respiratory syncytial virus (RSV). RSV is a major cause of childhood lung infections. Exposure to smoke increases the risk factor for RSV infections and hospitalization; and Stoddard and Aligne estimated that 25 percent of RSV infections were smoking-related. Current statistics show RSV infections cause 513 childhood deaths per year; therefore eliminating exposure to secondhand smoke could prevent 113 of those deaths.

Totaling these figures, we find that 4075 deaths each year would be prevented if parents did not smoke or allow their babies and children to be exposed to smoke. Unfortunately, some of these estimates are imprecise and no comprehensive studies of the childhood deaths due to smoking have been performed. Another way to estimate the deaths due to smoking is from compiled birth and death records from the states. With every birth certificate, data on the smoking habits of the mother is collected and death records can be linked to the birth record data.

Each year the CDC compiles these figures to follow trends in infant mortality. Analysis of childhood birth and death data reveals the infant mortality rate to be 60 to 70 percent higher in smoking mothers. The number of deaths attributed to smoking from these figures is 1932 deaths for the year 2001 and 2063 deaths in 2002. These figures look only at children who died in the first year of life and rely on the mother's self report of her smoking behavior. Studies that collected blood to compare directly measured nicotine levels to women's self-reported smoking histories found that as many as 25 percent of the studied women lie about their smoking behavior and underestimate the amount they smoke.

Causes of Death

The causes of death attributable to parental and secondhand smoke include:

SIDS (sudden infant death)	**585**
Low birth weight	**3100**
Lung infections and asthma	**140**
Fires	**250**
Total	**4075 deaths/year**

Figure 2.1 Table breaking down how smoking causes childhood deaths.

Smoking is responsible for more childhood deaths than...
Drowning, Fires, Accidents, or Poisoning,
Combined!

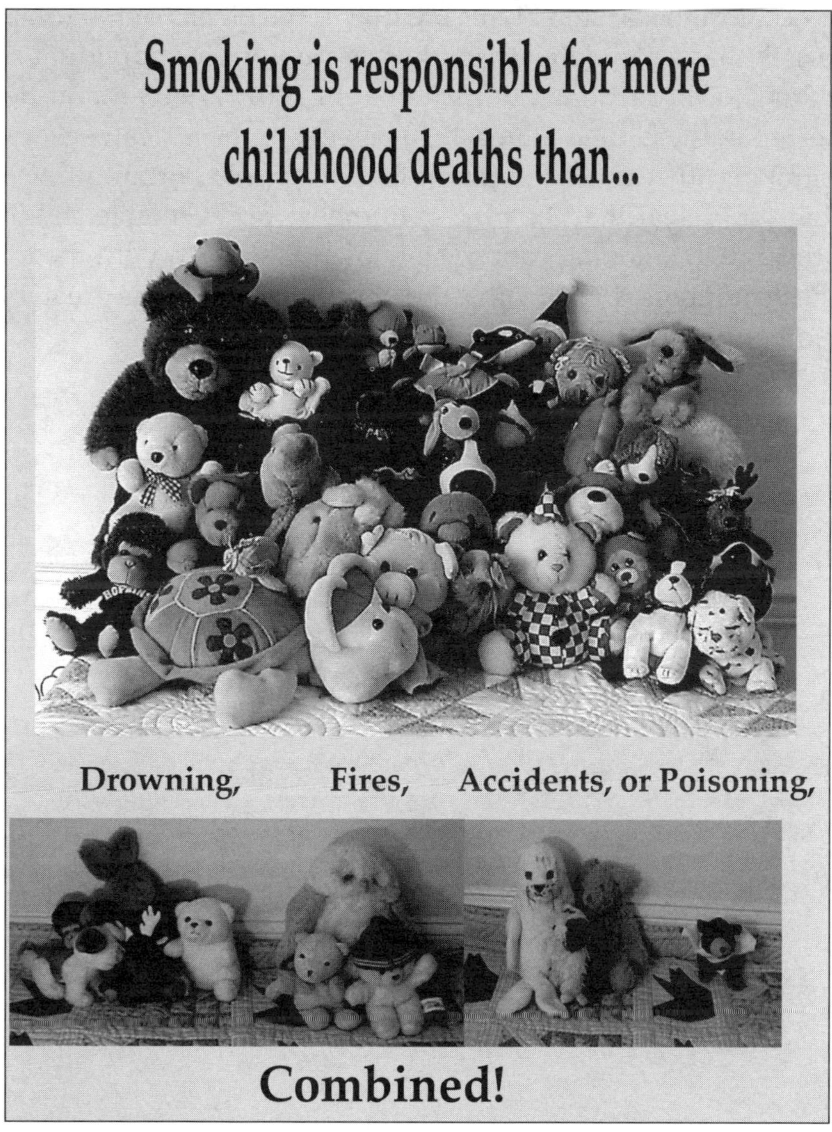

Figure 2.2 The photographs represent the children that die annually from preventable causes. Each stuffed animal stands for 100 children. The figures are 4100 for smoking, 520 for drowning, 270 for fires, 310 for car accidents, and 80 for poisoning.

The CDC has estimated that 10 percent of all infant deaths that occur in the United States are due to the effects of tobacco. This is largely based on detailed studies carried out in individual states such as North Carolina and Arizona. In 2001, 27,568 infant deaths occurred in the United States. If 10 percent of those deaths were due to smoking, this gives a number of 2756 deaths. From all of these studies, it is clear that the precise number of preventable childhood deaths due to smoking cannot be known. But, even with the lowest of these numbers, 1932 deaths, the impact of smoking is greater than any other preventable cause of childhood death.

Then...

"If we had any thought or knowledge that in any way we were selling a product harmful to consumers, we would stop business tomorrow."

- George Weissman, Vice President of Philip Morris, in 1954.

"If I saw or thought there were any evidence whatsoever that conclusively proved that, in some way, tobacco was harmful to people, and I believed in my heart and my soul, then I would get out of the business and I wouldn't be involved in it. Honestly I have not seen one piece of medical evidence that has been presented by anybody, anywhere that absolutely, totally said that smoking caused the disease or created it."

- Gerald H. Long, President of R.J. Reynolds, in 1986.

And Now...

"I have always believed that smoking plays a role in causing lung cancer."

- Steven F. Goldstone, Chairman of R.J.R.-Nabisco, in 1997.

Chapter 3. Before Birth

Cigarettes, Mother, and Baby

"Women who smoke like men, die like men"
- Dr. C. Everett Koop

Smoking and women's health

The early 1900s saw a great explosion in the use of tobacco. The invention of the tobacco-rolling machine allowed large quantities of cheap cigarettes to be produced. Cigarettes were given to soldiers fighting in World War I, and people at home were urged to send them to the men overseas. Upon their return, many soldiers were addicted to nicotine, and smoking was common. At the time, few women smoked. Those who did were seen as 'loose' or of 'poor breeding.' That thinking began to change in the 1920s with the increased influence of the women's rights movement. The 1920s were a time of greatly increased change for women and it became more socially acceptable for them to smoke. The tobacco companies took advantage of the opportunity. Ads began appearing targeting women, and new cigarettes were produced specifically to appeal to the 'fairer sex.' Cigarette smoking among women rose to 6 percent in 1924 and 12 percent in 1929.

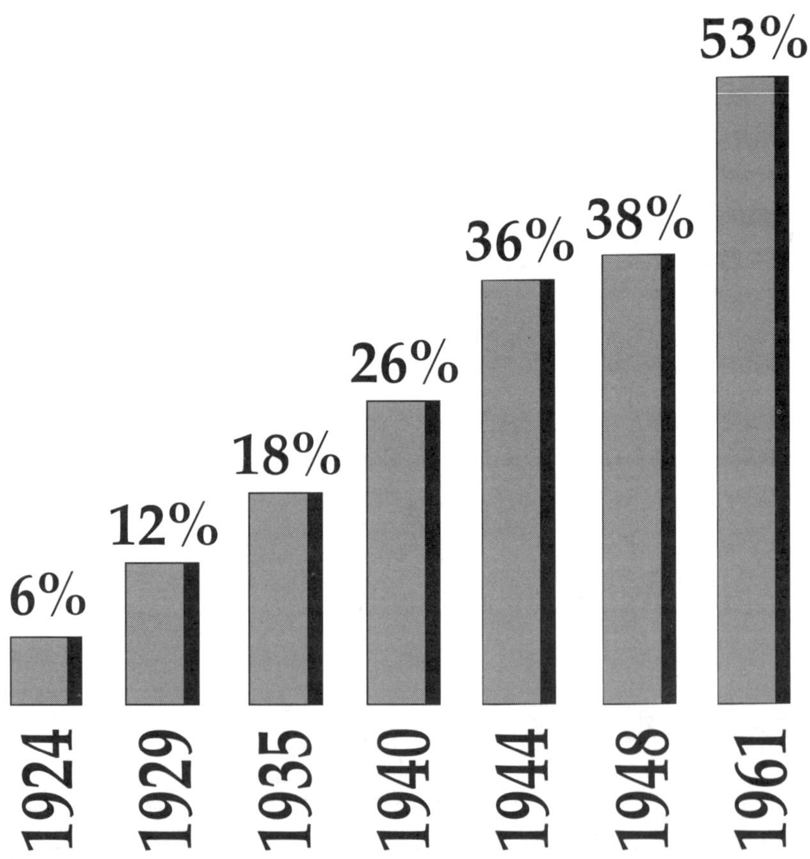

Figure 3.1 Proportion of adult female smokers.

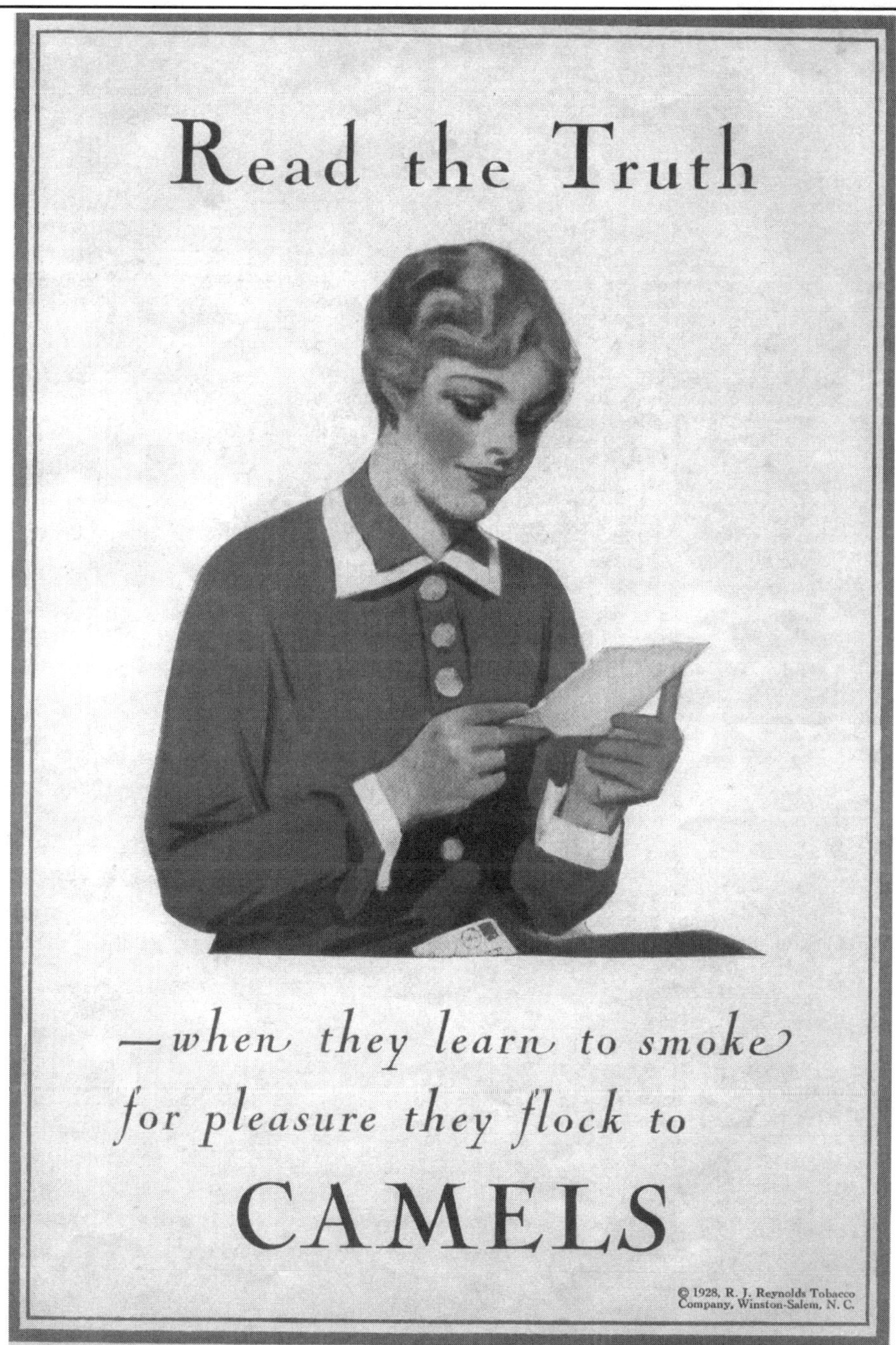

Figure 3.2 A 1920s Tobacco ad.

Watch the change to Chesterfield
says DONNA DAE
CHESTERFIELD'S JANUARY GIRL
starring with
FRED WARING'S PENNSYLVANIANS
Chesterfield
CIGARETTES
FORECASTING MORE SMOKING PLEASURE FOR 1940

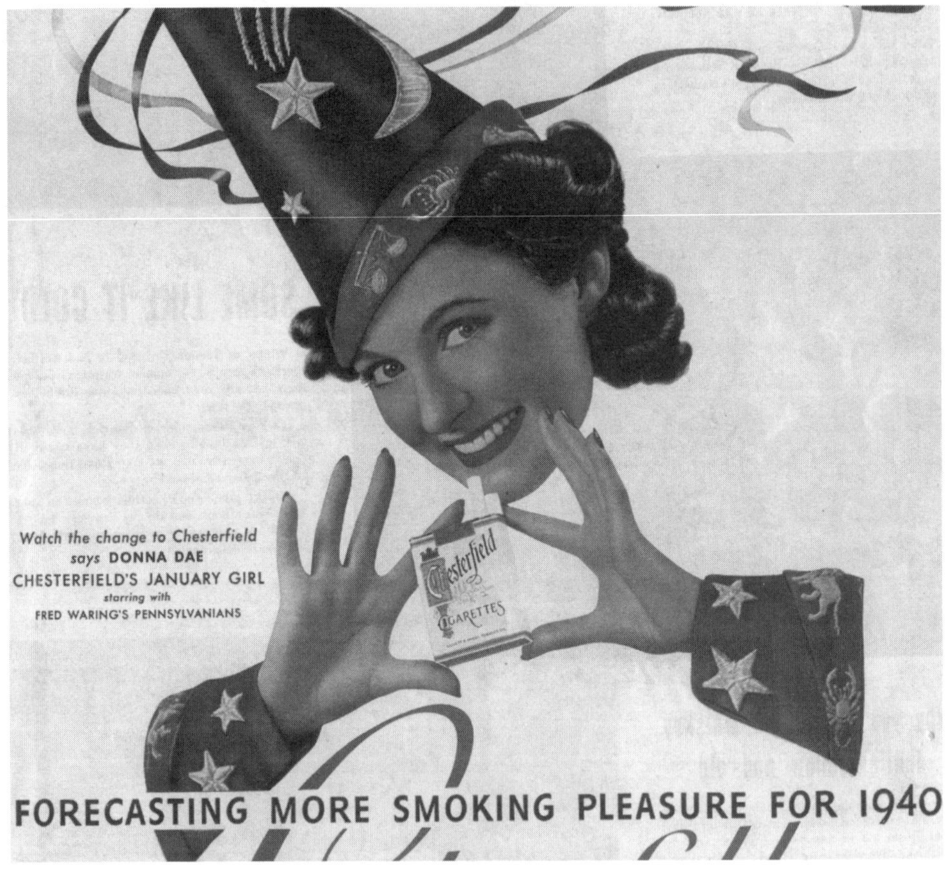

Figure 3.2 1940 Cigarette advertisement. Featuring Donna Dae "Chesterfield's January Girl".

During World War II, many women entered the work force for the first time, and with a large number of the men gone, social barriers to smoking were largely eliminated. In the United States, cigarette consumption more than doubled from 1935 to 1945, reaching 340 billion per year. The percentage of women who smoked rose to 26 percent in 1940 and to 36 percent in 1948.

Cigarette advertising kept pace with the changes in society. Women were prominently featured in tobacco ads, and products and marketing continued to be tailored to the male and female markets. Soon women had equality in smoking and began smoking just as much as men. The peak for female smoking rates is estimated to be 53 percent in 1961 and has since gradually declined to the current estimate of 20 percent.

In the beginning, women lagged behind men in displaying the health effects of smoking. On average, it takes thirty years for an increase in smoking to show up as an increase in deaths from lung cancer. In the figure below, you can see that lung cancer rates in males climbed rapidly starting in the 1930s and 1940s, reflecting the great increase in smoking at the turn of the century. In the 1940s, the first scientific studies began to be published showing a link between smoking and lung cancer. This line of studies culminated in the landmark 1964 United States Surgeon General's report on smoking. The increase in lung cancer for women did not begin until the 1970s. But, by the 1985-to-1989 time period, lung cancer overtook breast cancer as the number one cancer that was killing white females in the United States. And, after 1990, lung cancer became the largest cause of cancer deaths in African American women. Only in 2004 does there appear to be a leveling off of female lung cancer rates.

While there are more cases of breast cancer in women than lung cancer, lung cancer is more often fatal, and therefore the number of deaths due to lung cancer is higher. In fact, lung cancer kills more Americans than breast cancer, prostate cancer, colon cancer, liver cancer, kidney cancer, and skin cancer - combined. While lung cancer primarily afflicts smokers and former smokers, there is a disturbing

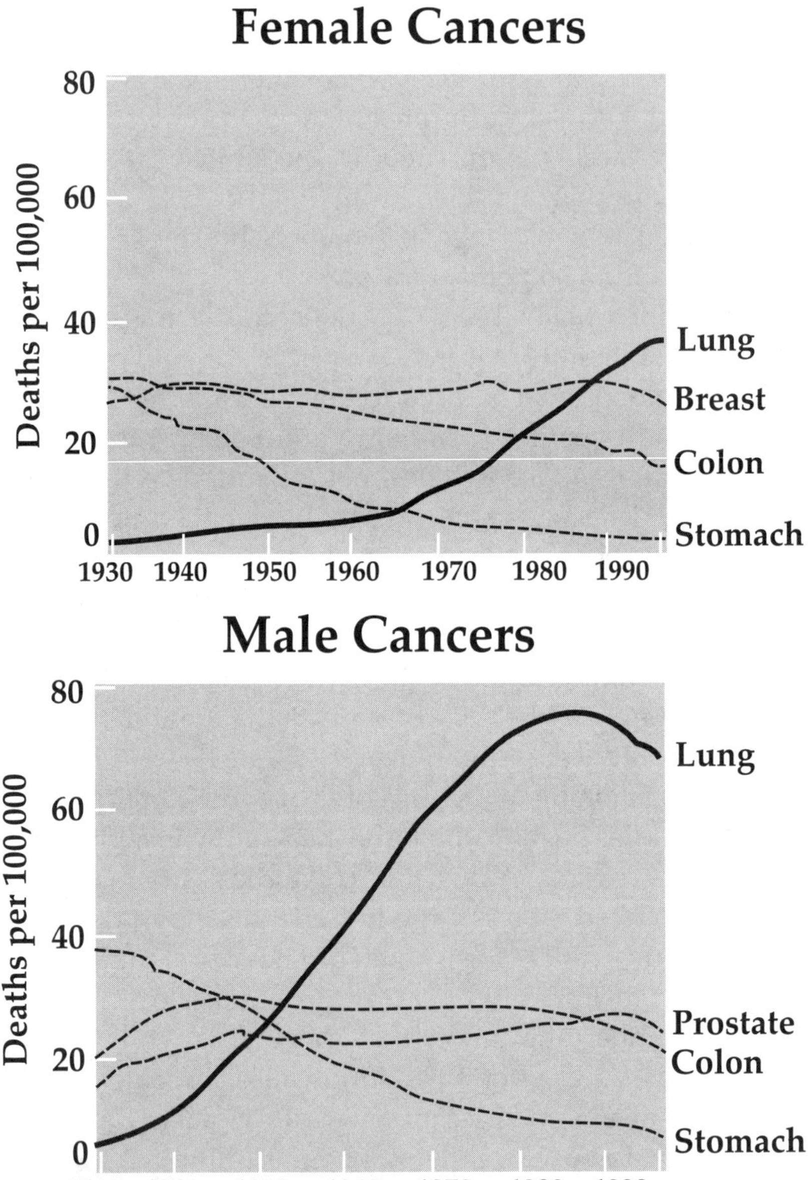

Figure 3.3 Death rates from the major cancers in males and females from the years 1930 to 2000. Lung cancer became the number one killer of men in the 1950s and of females in the 1980s.

trend of lung tumors appearing in younger, nonsmoking women. Dana Reeve is only the most visible new victim. Dana, the wife of Christopher Reeve, was a nonsmoker who died of lung cancer in 2006 at the age of 44.

An explanation for the apparent rise in lung cancer among nonsmokers is still lacking. "Many of them have done an excellent job of taking care of themselves," said Dr. Joan Schiller, who specializes in lung cancer in nonsmoking younger women at the University of Wisconsin in Madison. "They run. They eat right" (http://www.lungcanceralliance.org/). While the cause of the cancer in these women cannot be known, secondhand smoke is a known risk factor for lung cancer.

Smoking and Reproductive Health

While lung cancer is the most deadly outcome of smoking, tobacco use causes a whole range of reproductive problems and diseases in both men and women. Reports by the United States Surgeon General's office and the British Medical Association have compiled data from many scientific studies to back up these findings. The good news is that quitting smoking can reverse most of the damage and reduce the risk of disease.

Smoking affects all aspects of reproduction. Women who smoke have a significantly lower fertility rate, a higher risk of miscarriage, and experience many other complications of pregnancy. This is powerful evidence of the profound effect of tobacco smoke on female health. Smoking affects the breakdown of estrogens in a woman's body as well as affecting male sex hormones. Therefore smoking is said to have an 'antiestrogenic' effect. The consequence of this antiestrogen effect is a decreased rate of fertility and an earlier entry into menopause. Women who smoke are also more likely to develop a male-type distribution of body fat, with more fat located in the stomach area and less in the hips. Fat distribution is in part determined by sex hormones. The effect of smoking on estrogen breakdown means smoking can also affect synthetic estrogens present in birth control

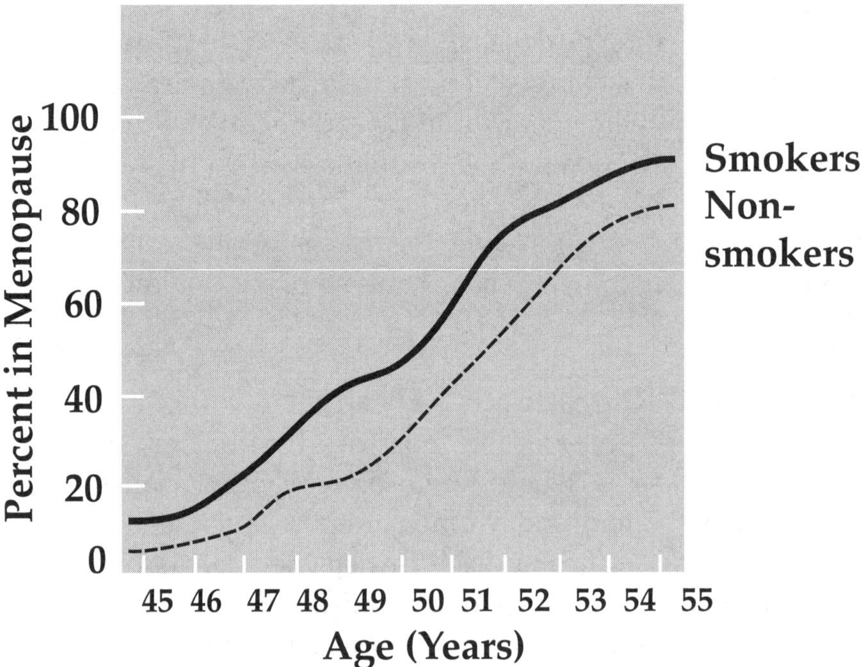

Figure 3.5 Earlier menopause in smokers. The entry of women into menopause begins in the 40s and increases to nearly 100 percent by age 65. At all ages smokers have a greater chance of being menopausal. This is due to the estrogen inhibiting properties of smoking.

pills. Smoking women are twice as likely to experience a failure of the pill and an unwanted pregnancy. Tobacco use and the estrogen-containing pill combine to greatly increase a woman's risk of stroke and heart disease. Some studies show that women on the pill who smoke have a risk of heart disease twenty times than women on the pill alone. Women smokers also have a lower risk of endometrial cancer, a cancer that is dependent on estrogen.

Smoking also dramatically affects male reproduction. Male smokers experience a higher incidence of impotence, a lower sperm count and a higher proportion of malformed sperm. The combined effects on male and female fertility reduce the ability of smoking parents to conceive a child. A study of almost eleven thousand women in Denmark found that women who smoked between five and nine cigarettes a day were 1.8 times more likely than nonsmokers to fail to conceive within twelve months. Couples being treated for infertility have a poorer response to treatment if they smoke. Smoking women produce fewer eggs when stimulated by hormones, and the more they smoke, the fewer eggs they make. *In vitro* fertilization is less effective in smoking couples. If the male smokes, intracytoplasmic sperm injection (when sperm is artificially introduced into an egg) fails four out of five times.

Tobacco exposure dramatically affects the unborn child. Mothers who smoke have more spontaneous abortions or miscarriages. The most reliable data on this come from studies of mothers undergoing *in vitro* fertilization where both the number of implanted embryos and the number of successful pregnancies are known. In one of these studies, 42 percent of smoking mothers miscarried compared to 19 percent of nonsmoking mothers. From this data, one can estimate that a great many miscarriages in the United States are due to smoking. Many of these miscarriages are likely to occur early in the pregnancy and go unnoticed. One study, published in the *Journal of Family Practice,* estimated that smoking caused from 19 to 140 thousand spontaneous abortions per year.

However this figure has been questioned, and the true number is hard to determine accurately.

Stillbirth, ectopic pregnancy, and premature delivery happen more often in mothers who smoke. Smoking mothers also have higher rates of placenta previa (placenta blocking the cervix), a dangerous complication of pregnancy, and placental abruption, where the placenta tears away from the uterus. Both of these conditions can lead to serious consequences, including death for both mother and unborn child.

While cigarette smoke contains many harmful chemicals, nicotine itself is capable of causing birth defects. Nicotine works by binding to receptors in the brain that normally respond to the signaling molecule acetylcholine. Exposure of the developing embryo to nicotine can lead to abnormal amounts and distribution of these receptors, causing developmental abnormalities. Studies by the CDC have associated nicotine exposure to such behavioral disorders in children and adolescents as attention deficit/hyperactivity disorder and impaired performances on standardized tests and in school. While these behavioral studies are hard to carry out and are not conclusive, they provide yet another justification for reducing or eliminating tobacco exposure to infants and children.

Many government programs are in place to reduce infant mortality and increase childhood safety. Most states require infants and children to ride in approved child car seats and strictly regulate cribs, toys, and appliances. It is therefore strange that we have placed relatively little attention on preventable deaths caused by tobacco. The massive advertising and lobbying budgets of the tobacco industry certainly play a role in suppressing the information on the dangers to children of smoking, and these companies persistently fight stricter measures to limit smoking in public places. However, by focusing on child safety, we can reduce childhood exposure to tobacco smoke and improve child health.

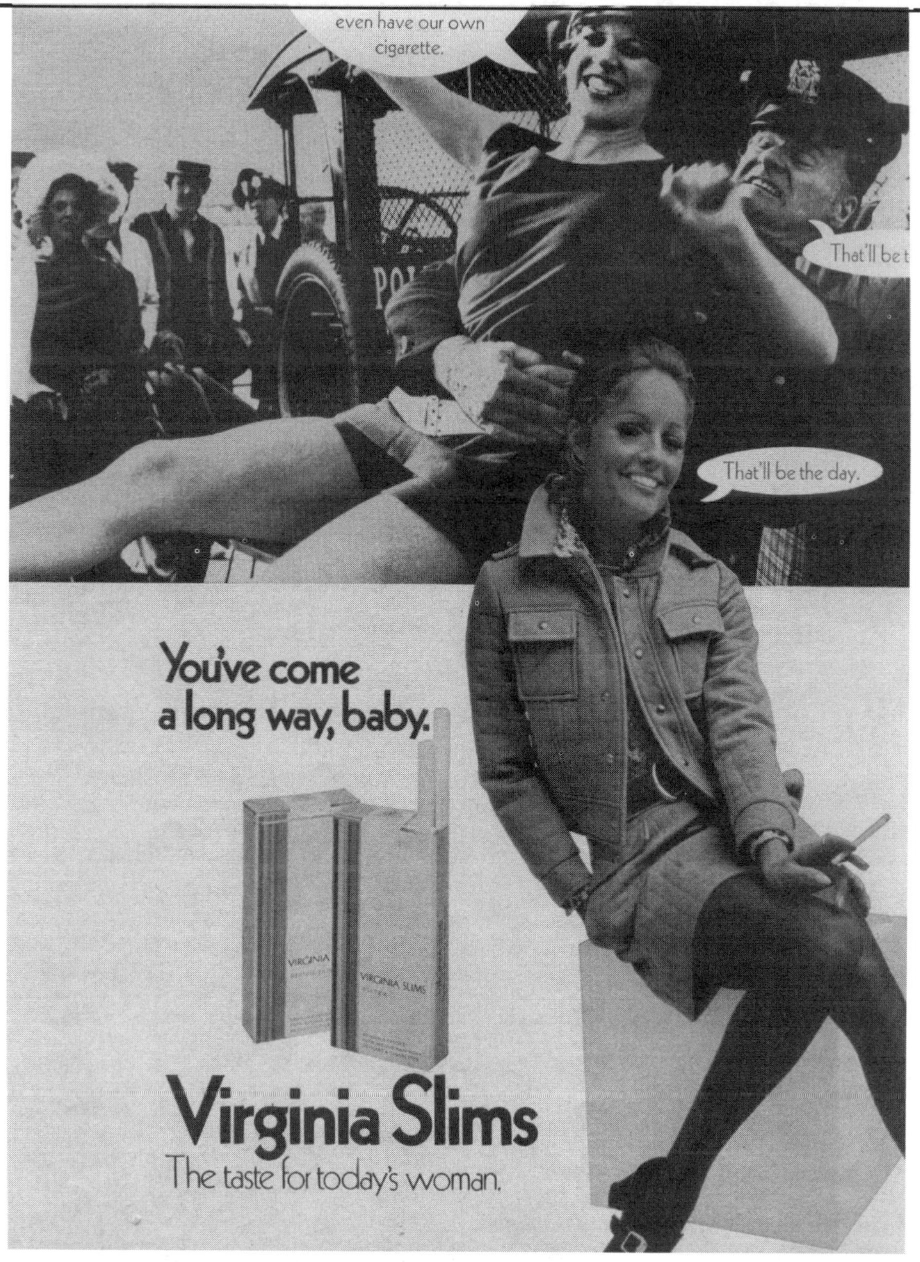

Figure 3.4 You HAVE come a long way! Upper caption reads "You just wait! Someday we'll be able to wear any bathing suit we want, Someday we'll be able to vote. Someday we'll be able to smoke just like a man. Someday we'll even have our own cigarette."

What can you do?

- If you are a woman who is pregnant or planning to have a child, stop smoking now.
- Insist on a strictly smoke-free environment for your baby including your home, transportation, restaurants, and childcare.
- Help educate parents and prospective parents about the dangers tobacco smoke poses to children.
- Health care providers should more proactively deliver the latest information to patients and parents.
- Lobby your local and national elected representatives for better health care for women.

Part II. The Solutions

Chapter 4 Healthy Mothers, Healthy Babies

Five Ways to Prevent Infant Death

The health of a woman who is pregnant is obviously critical to insure a healthy baby. Humans are amazingly resilient, and healthy babies have been born to mothers who have survived deplorable conditions. However, scientists have discovered that the health of the mother profoundly affects the health of her children — and even her grandchildren. One of these studies followed children born to mothers who became pregnant during the terrible famine that occurred in the Netherlands during World War II. Not only did the children of these mothers have an increased incidence of health problems, but there were also health problems observed in their grandchildren. Dietary excesses or restrictions in mice and monkeys also affect not only the offspring of the mother but also the offspring born in the next generation.

A number of infectious diseases such as rubella (German measles), syphilis, and cytomegalovirus cause birth defects in the children of infected mothers. Similarly certain drugs such as thalidomide and Accutane, if taken during pregnancy, cause developmental abnormalities to occur, as does exposure to radiation and toxins. Obesity and diabetes in the pregnant mother increase the risk of disease in her children. While the influence of maternal health on childhood diseases is relatively easy to document, there is also evidence that later onset conditions — like adult diabetes, obesity, high blood pressure, and heart disease — are also influenced by the health and nutrition of the mother.

Deficiencies in vitamins and minerals also lead to an increased incidence of certain conditions, such as neural tube defects. Therefore, it is very important to ensure that pregnant women are given the very best nutrition and medical care, and are protected from environmental poisons.

Here are five ways that a woman can improve the health of her baby

- Do not smoke or have excessive exposure to tobacco smoke, and don't drink alcohol.
- Take a multivitamin, particularly one with four hundred micrograms of folic acid
- Have a regular exercise program with a minimum of thirty minutes of walking (for as long as you are able and after consultation with your doctor).
- Eat a healthy diet — rich in fruits and vegetables and low in fat.
- Get regular prenatal medical care.

Following these simple guidelines will result in a dramatically reduced risk of such diseases in the mother as gestational diabetes, increase the chance of normal birth weight of the infant, and decrease the risks of mental retardation and birth defects.

The Planning Problem

Many of the factors affecting the health of the baby are most critical during the first three months of pregnancy. During this period, the fetus is growing very quickly, and many organs of the body are developing. Therefore, proper nutrition and protection of the mother from infections and toxins before pregnancy are critical. However, many pregnancies are unplanned. In fact, of the more than four million births occurring in the United States every year, about half are not planned, and the rate is even greater in individuals at high risk for poor pregnancy outcomes.

For this reason, it is critical to improve the health and medical care of all women of childbearing age. Of course all of the guidelines given above are good advice for any of us, male or female.

Smoking and Drinking

Both tobacco and alcohol consumed by the mother are harmful to the developing baby, but in different ways. Smoking results in the delivery to the baby, through the mother's blood, of nicotine along with many other harmful chemicals. Probably the most harmful such chemical is carbon monoxide, the same poisonous gas that comes out of the exhaust pipe of your car. This poison attaches to the hemoglobin protein found in red blood cells, the molecule that delivers oxygen from the mother's lungs to the baby.

Carbon monoxide replaces the oxygen in red blood cells and robs hemoglobin of the ability to do its job. The result is oxygen deprivation. This oxygen starvation is thought to be a major cause of the lower birth weight of babies born to smoking or smoke-exposed mothers. Nicotine itself is classified as a developmental toxin, because scientific studies show that it causes fetal abnormalities. Other toxins such as lead, cadmium, cyanide, and benzene are also found in tobacco smoke, and all are dangerous to the baby.

Studies of mothers who smoked different amounts of cigarettes during pregnancy demonstrate that there is no safe level of smoking. Children born to heavy smokers have a higher rate of SIDS and infant mortality than do light smokers, but light smokers have a higher incidence than nonsmokers. Quitting smoking at any time during pregnancy benefits the baby, and the earlier the mother quits, the better.

Excessive drinking of any alcoholic beverage during pregnancy is known to harm babies. The poor outcomes include lower birth weight, mental retardation, abnormal facial features, birth defects, and behavioral or learning problems. This combination of symptoms is known as fetal alcohol syndrome or fetal alcohol abuse syndrome. The alcohol a mother drinks passes directly into the blood of the growing baby, altering normal development of the face, heart, bones, eyes, and ears. Brain scans of babies suffering from fetal alcohol abuse syndrome show abnormalities in the function of the developing brain. The severity of these effects depends on the amount of drinking, the time during pregnancy when the exposure happens, as well as other nutritional and genetic factors. However, there is no known safe level of exposure and the early weeks are the most critical. "We must prevent all injury and illness that is preventable in society, and alcohol-related birth defects are completely preventable", says United Stated Surgeon General Richard H. Carmona. **Women who are pregnant or plan to become pregnant should avoid all smoking and exposure to smoke and should refrain from any drinking.**

Vitamins and folic acid

Proper nutrition of the mother during pregnancy is critical to the development of the baby. Particularly important are several vitamins and minerals. For this reason pregnant women are given a daily prenatal vitamin. Although many vitamins and minerals can be obtained from a balanced diet, it is best to ensure that the full requirements are met. Folic acid, one of the B vitamins, is needed for the synthesis of DNA and is critical to the growing baby. Women

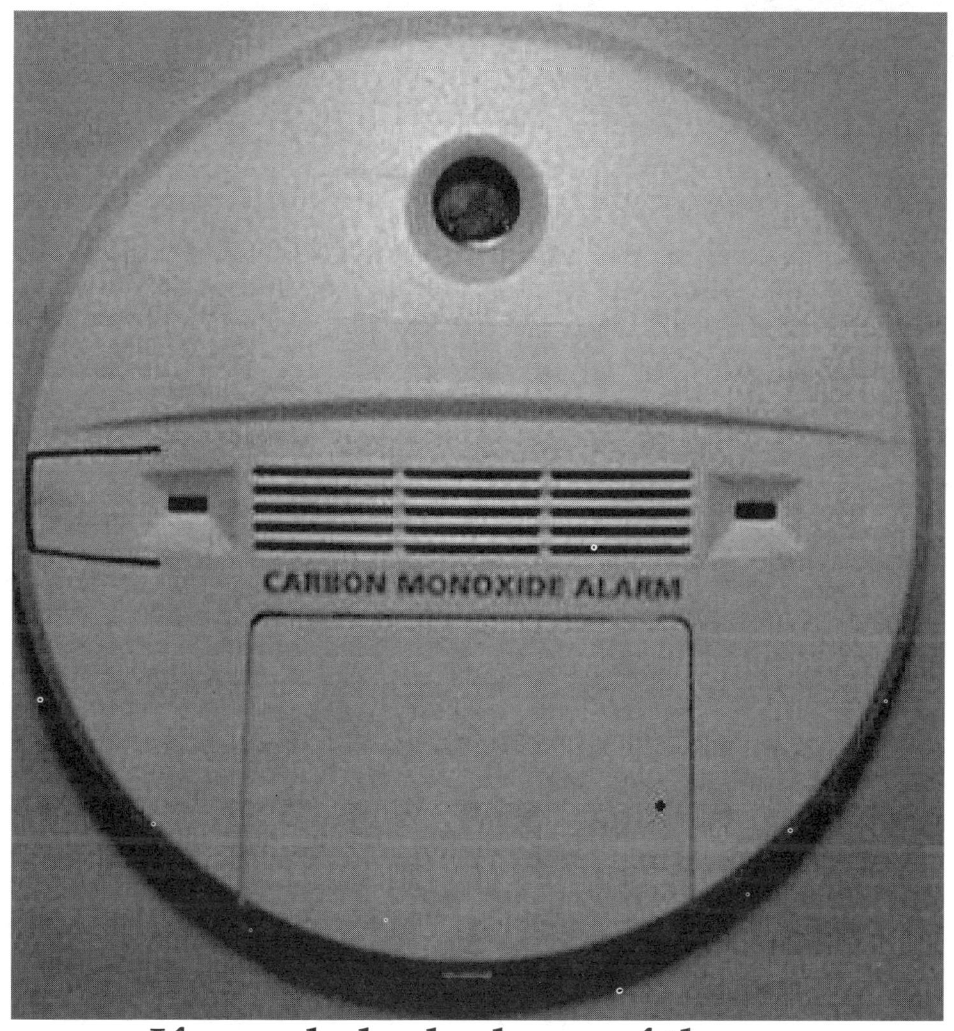

If your baby had one of these...

It would go off every time you smoke!

Figure 4.1 Carbon Monoxide detector. Smoking mothers inhale the poison carbon monoxide, leading to oxygen starvation of the baby.

with a folic acid deficiency run a greater risk of having a baby with cleft lip, cleft palate and certain brain and spine development defects such as spina bifida. These classes of birth defects are known as neural tube defects. Women pregnant with twins, or with a family history of neural tube defects may be prescribed additional folic acid.

Women also need extra calcium during pregnancy to help build the baby's bones. Doctors recommend that pregnant women eat four servings a day of dairy foods. Greens, broccoli, calcium-fortified orange juice, and tortillas are other good calcium sources. Women also need extra iron in the last six months of the pregnancy to help produce additional red blood cells and to grow the baby's placenta. The prenatal vitamins satisfy most women's iron needs. The Women, Infants, and Children (WIC) program provides nutritional assistance to low-income pregnant women and their children up to age five (http://www.fns.usda.gov/wic). This program has been effective at reducing infant mortality and reducing health care costs.

Exercise

Maintaining physical fitness is critical to pregnant women for many reasons. Getting to a healthy weight before pregnancy can mean an easier time becoming pregnant and an easier pregnancy. Following a regular diet and exercise plan helps a woman gain the proper amount of weight during pregnancy, ensuring a healthy birth weight for the baby. A physically fit woman is better able to handle the demands of the late stages of pregnancy and delivery. Lastly, exercise helps to relieve stress.

A doctor or other health care provider should approve all exercise programs. Most women can continue their normal exercise regimen. The American College of Obstetricians and Gynecologists recommends thirty minutes or more of moderate exercise per day for healthy pregnant women. Walking, swimming, aerobic exercise, weight training, and yoga are all good choices. Doctors recommend against dangerous and contact sports — in fact, any activity that could result in trauma to the abdomen. Scuba diving and high altitude

If you are pregnant, you can safely drink ...

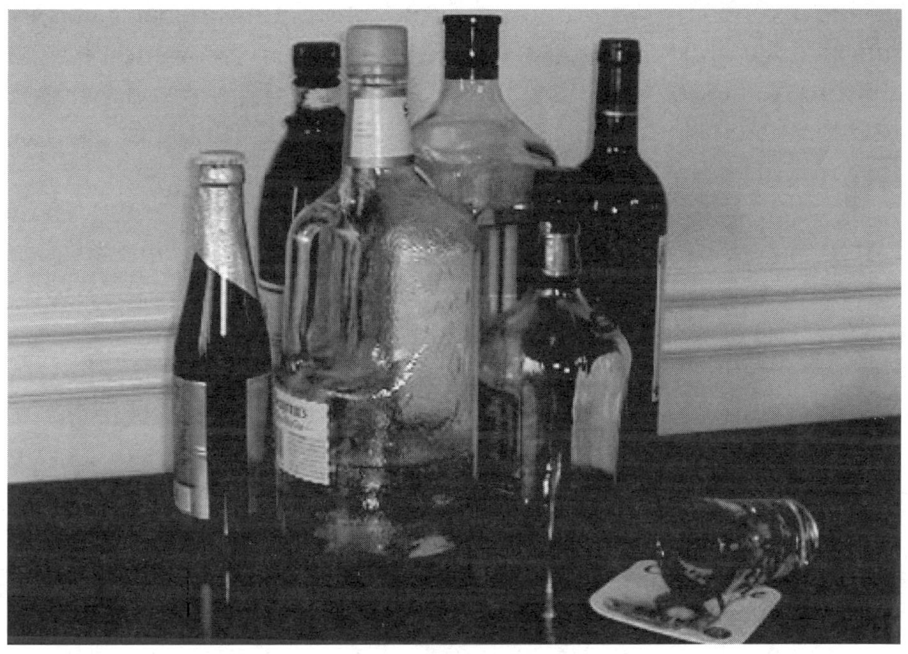

Nothing!

The Surgeon General says that there is no safe level of alcohol for your baby. So wait until after your healthy child is born to celebrate!

Figure 4.2 Alcohol and Pregnancy. Current recommendations say there is no safe level of drinking during pregnancy.

sports are also forbidden. Late in pregnancy, exercises involving lying flat on the back are not recommended, as blood flow to the mother or the baby could be restricted.

Avoid exercising on an empty stomach. Eating a snack and/or drinking juice thirty minutes before exercise is recommended to maintain your blood sugar levels. Exercisers should stay hydrated by drinking a cup of water before exercising and another cup every twenty minutes during exercise.

Healthy Diet

A healthy diet during pregnancy helps insure a healthy newborn. The best success comes to women who are a healthy weight before pregnancy. Typically, a woman requires three hundred extra calories per day during pregnancy to achieve her target weight gain. However, morning sickness, and food aversions and cravings can make this difficult to achieve. The amount of weight a woman should gain depends on her weight at the start of pregnancy. Underweight women — those with a body mass index (BMI) below 20 — should gain twenty-eight to forty pounds, while those at a normal weight (BMI= 20 to 26) should gain twenty-five to thirty-five pounds. Overweight women (BMI = 26 to 29) should gain fifteen to twenty-five pounds, and obese women fifteen pounds.

The ideal diet should include fruits and vegetables, grains, beans, and low-fat meats. Vegetarian diets can be followed if particular attention is paid to obtaining sufficient complete protein, vitamins, and minerals. Foods not recommended include uncooked deli meats, raw or undercooked meats, fish, or eggs, because of the danger from bacterial and viral infection. Several infections, such as *Salmonella*, other bacteria, and viruses, are harmful to the unborn, and efforts should be made to avoid them.

Controversy exists about the danger of mercury in fish. On the one hand, the fats found in many fish are beneficial to fetal development. On the other, mercury exposure in animals can cause damage to developing brains, resulting in learning disabilities and hearing loss. However, documenting these effects in people has been difficult. Foods potentially high in mercury include most large fish such as swordfish and sharks, as well as local wild fish, including trout, bass, and salmon. Current guidelines recommend eating no more than six ounces of albacore (white) tuna or tuna steak each week.

A number of excellent resources are available for women to consult. The March of Dimes (www.marchofdimes.com) provides information on ways to ensure a healthy child and suggests steps to take before and during pregnancy. The Women, Infants, and Children (WIC) program (www.fns.usda.gov/wic) provides prenatal nutrition for pregnant mothers and nutritional support and immunizations for children under five years old. Babyfit.com (www.babyfit.com) provides recipes and exercise programs and other resources free to interested individuals.

Medical Care

Increasing access to and use of medical care for women of childbearing age will improve the health of babies in the United States. Many of the problems leading to infant mortality can be avoided through better health care. This includes improved nutrition, immunization, and education for women who might become pregnant, as well as better care of women during pregnancy. The most underserved populations of women, those with the highest incidence of infant mortality, are white women who did not finish high school, African American women, and Native Americans. Each of these populations has a higher rate of poverty, a lower rate of coverage by health insurance, and reduced access to medical care.

Such untreated medical problems as diabetes, heart conditions, autoimmune disease, liver or kidney disease, obesity, infections, and high blood pressure can lead to complications during pregnancy. Common problems in pregnancy include preeclampsia (high blood pressure and toxemia), gestational diabetes, asthma, urinary infections, and anemia. Poor medical care during pregnancy can lead to postpartum (after birth) infections, hemorrhage (severe bleeding), and depression. Preeclampsia alone affects about 5 to 10 percent of all pregnancies and is found most often in very young mothers and in those of advanced age. Preeclampsia is one of the leading causes of death of pregnant women and of their babies. While the causes are complex, if recognized early, preeclampsia can be effectively treated.

African American women have by far the highest rate of death during pregnancy and delivery of any group (two to three times as high as Hispanic, Asian and Native Americans and four times higher than whites). Hypertension is particularly common in African American women and is the source of a large number of complications during pregnancy. Women with sickle cell trait have an increased risk of anemia and urinary tract infections. Diabetes is also a common complication in both African and Native American women and if untreated can be an important cause of pregnancy complications. Asian and Hispanic descent is a risk factor for postpartum hemorrhage, an important cause of maternal death.

Reducing infant mortality and complications during pregnancy remain some of the most challenging medical problems facing our country. The causes are complex, and solutions require multiple approaches. Improving the health care of all women, particularly in underserved areas, is the most effective solution. In addition, education is of vital importance, as a great many problems can be reduced or eliminated by providing families and communities with the information that they need to reduce the health problems causing infant mortality. Healthy choices in lifestyle, diet, stress management, and exercise are of critical importance to women who are pregnant or that may become pregnant.

Chapter 5. Money Talks

Consumer Strategies to Combat Cigarette Tobacco Use

Effectively tackling the problem of smoking and childhood tobacco-related disease will require considerable effort by individuals to bring about change and improve education. Citizens concerned about the impact of tobacco can lobby political leaders to change governmental policies. However, the power of consumers is enormous and has not been fully applied to the problem of tobacco addiction in children and young people. Economic pressures and public opinion have resulted in changes for other social and health causes. Activists succeeded in getting greater access to therapies for AIDS and breast cancer, and economic pressure has helped bring about social change in the United States and elsewhere.

A campaign to reduce infant nicotine exposure, and childhood smoking and tobacco addiction, should be relatively free of controversy. We have laws banning the sale of tobacco products to children, yet we expose them to considerable tobacco advertising as well as tobacco use in movies and other media. We allow the sale of tobacco products in stores that children frequent and all too many preteens and teens have access to tobacco products in their homes.

Sweden became the first country to reduce cigarette smoking to below 20 percent of the adult population. They achieved this through a program which combined tobacco education, innovative tobacco cessation programs, and restrictions on advertising. Sweden also became one of several European countries to ban smoking in the workplace. "I don't think anyone believes that the right of smokers to smoke is more important than the right for everyone to breath fresh air," says Margaretha Haglund, head of tobacco control programs at the Swedish National Institute of Public Health (www.sweden.se). However, Sweden has a particularly high incidence of the use of smokeless tobacco, a health problem in its own right.

Magazines and Tobacco Advertising

To survive, the tobacco companies need new cigarette smokers. Many adults eventually quit smoking, and those consumers need to be replaced with new ones. The tobacco companies attract new smokers through a $15.2 billion marketing budget. This advertising goal is to increase smoking in young people because very few people start smoking or change brands after the age of twenty-one. The ads clearly work as nearly all underage smokers use one of the three most heavily advertised brands. Therefore, reducing the exposure of children to tobacco ads is an effective way to combat underage smoking.

In 2004 and 2005, cigarette ads were placed in thirty-six major magazines with a combined circulation of over 50 million copies. Three to five other people read each copy of these magazines, which means that these advertisements reach nearly the entire country. Some of the most popular publications, found in nearly every household, such as *People, Time, Sports Illustrated,* and *Newsweek,* contain tobacco ads. There are magazines for girls and young women

State Cigarette Taxes

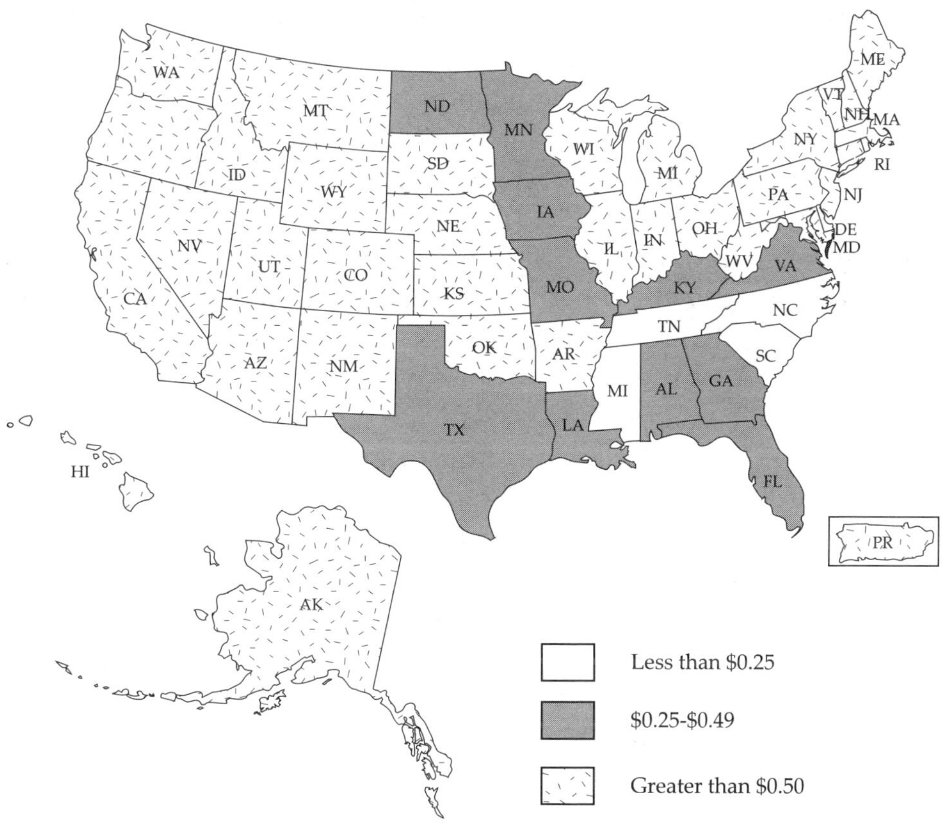

Figure 5.1 Map of State Cigarette Taxes. States with taxes of more than $0.50 per pack are shown in grey, $0.25-0.50 per pack are strippled, and less than $0.25 per pack in white.

(*Cosmopolitan, Vogue, Lucky*), for boys and young men (*Car and Driver, FHM, Maxim*), for music fans (*Rolling Stone, Blender, Tracks*), and for African Americans and Hispanics (*Ebony, Essence, Latina, People en Español*).

True, many of the magazines target an adult audience. Over 70 percent of the women who buy *Cosmopolitan* are over twenty-four as are 60 percent of the men that buy *Maxim*. But the target audience for the cigarette ads is the under-eighteen crowd that gets a hold of these forbidden publications (I was ten when I found my father's *Playboy* collection). Preteens and teens want to be independent and self-confident. For the tobacco industry, the beauty of ads in adult publications is that young people seek them out; they are "forbidden fruit."

Through magazines, cigarette ads are delivered to the school. Up until 2003, tobacco ads were found in specially prepared classroom editions of *Time* and *Newsweek* read by over one million students. This practice was discontinued under an agreement between the magazines, the advertisers, and the Attorney Generals of several states. However, many schools also subscribe to the regular editions of these magazines. A study by the New York State Department of Health determined that over 70 percent of the libraries in New York middle schools and high schools had copies of *Time, Newsweek, People* and *Sports Illustrated* containing cigarette ads. This led to a second agreement to remove the tobacco ads from the regular editions of these magazines before they get to the schools. This will reduce the exposure of children to tobacco ads at school, but the magazines in their homes will still contain tobacco ads.

Twenty publishers produce the thirty-six major magazines carrying cigarette ads, but three of these publishers account for half of the magazines. The Hearst Corporation produces seven of the magazines directly or through its affiliate iVillage. The iVillage company maintains a web site focused on topics of interest to women, with links to the web sites of *Cosmopolitan, Redbook, Marie Claire,* and other magazines. They also run the gURL site for teenage girls. Time

Warner is the company reaching the most households with smoking ads, through the publication of *Time, Sports Illustrated, People* and *Entertainment Weekly*. These publications have a combined circulation of over twelve million. Advance Publications, Inc., is a privately held company that includes CondeNast. It puts out a large number of magazines, mostly focused on women and fashion. Parents, of course, can choose whether or not to have these publications in the home. If exposing their children to tobacco ads concerns them, they can choose to stop buying these magazines or tear out the tobacco ads.

The tobacco companies have always relied heavily on advertising to push their products. The ban on advertising tobacco on TV and on most billboards has sent tobacco companies to newspapers and magazines. Tobacco is a legal product for adults; and publications exclusively read by adults, it can be argued, should be able to accept this advertising. However, minors also see many adult publications and other general interest publications containing tobacco ads. Most print publications depend on advertising to survive, so each publication balances the needs of their business with the needs of their readers. But many magazines and newspapers selling tobacco ads also have a mission to educate their readers on issues such as health and disease. Such publications have at least the appearance of a **conflict of interest** by accepting these ads.

In the year 2000, the major tobacco companies, agreed to stop advertising in magazines and newspapers read by over two million minors or whose readership was over 15 percent young people. This finally removed tobacco ads from some widely read publications. But the tobacco companies increased their advertising in magazines just below the two million and 15 percent limits and increased other forms of advertising.

A number of publications have taken a leadership role in refusing tobacco ads.

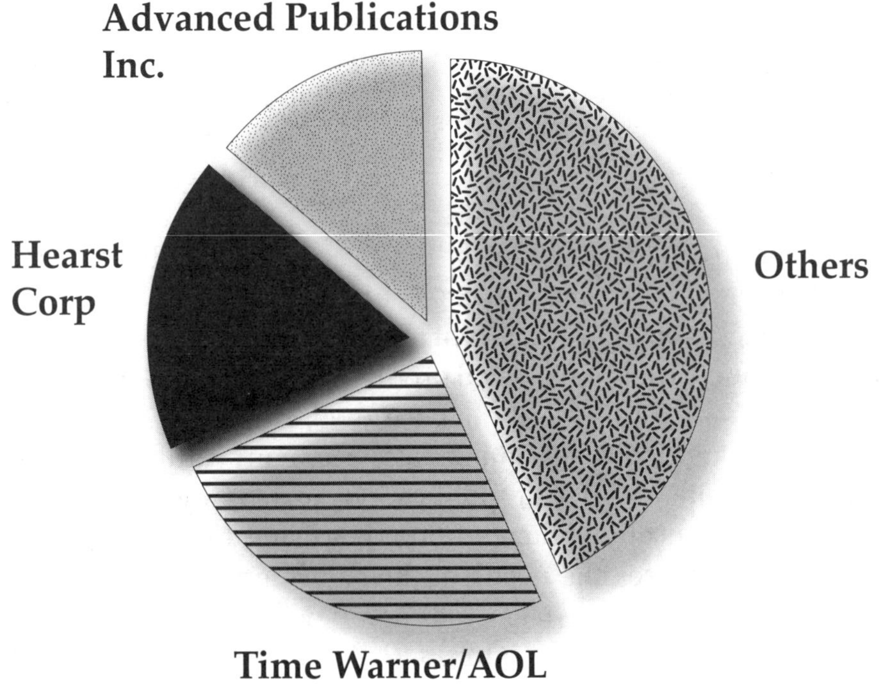

Figure 5.2 Three publishers account for over half of the magazines published with tobacco advertising. They are the Time Warner Corporation, The Hearst Corporation, and the privately held firm, Advanced Publications, Inc.

Reader's Digest began refusing tobacco advertising in 1924 and started publishing articles critical of smoking as early as 1941. Their 1952 article, "Cancer by the Carton" was one of the first articles to bring the connection between smoking and malignancy to the general public. *Good Housekeeping* has a long history of endorsing products which are pure and healthful (with the famous *Good Housekeeping Seal of Approval*). They employed Dr. Harvey Wiley in 1914, the founding director of the Food and Drug Administration (FDA). In 1927, Dr. Wiley began publishing articles on the potential unhealthful effects of smoking and of a connection to cancer. *Good Housekeeping* began in 1952 refusing to publish ads for tobacco products and has continued to publish articles on smoking and its effects on health.

In 1999, two of the largest newspapers in the country *The New York Times* and *The Boston Globe,* announced that they would no longer accept tobacco ads. "However, even though tobacco remains legal, its effect on public health is clear. We can no longer justify carrying advertisements that promote a product when the harm it causes is so evident and is now acknowledged even by one of the major tobacco companies," said *Globe* publisher Richard H. Gilman in a press release. "Our overall approach is to keep our pages — news, editorial and advertising — as open as we can. But given the effect of tobacco on the human body, we could not, in good conscience, continue to accept such advertising," says Arthur Sulzberger Jr., chairman of The New York Times Company and publisher of *The New York Times.*

These papers join a growing list of newspapers that refuse tobacco ads including *The Christian Science Monitor, San Jose Mercury News, Seattle Times,* and *Honolulu Star-Bulletin. The New York Times,* in particular, has produced strong investigative reporting on tobacco issues. Science and Health reporter Philip Hilts produced many ground-breaking stories on the tobacco industry and detailed these in his book, *Smokescreen: The Truth Behind the Tobacco Industry Cover-Up.*

The best source for information on tobacco advertising in magazines can be found at http://www.tobaccofreeperiodicals.org/. The site is maintained by the Maryland State Medical Society (MedChi) and several other medical and anti-tobacco organizations. At the site, ads for tobacco products as well as informational ads by the tobacco companies are tracked. MedChi opposes the presence of tobacco advertising in patient waiting areas, and so they maintain a list of tobacco-ad-free magazines and publications for the benefit of their members. The MedChi list contains over 100 magazines without ads, including *Better Homes and Gardens, Consumer Reports, Discover, National Geographic, House Beautiful, Men's Health, Ms., PC World, Saturday Evening Post, Scientific American,* and *Smithsonian.*

Some publications do not publish ads for tobacco products but print advertisements from tobacco companies presenting their views on smoking and health, or underage smoking. These public relations ads are controversial and typically portray smoking as a strictly adult activity. Studies show that these public relations ads are not effective at discouraging children from smoking. *The New York Times,* for example, allows such ads as they fall in the category of paid editorials, and similar ads appear in *Consumer's Digest, Forbes, The New Yorker, Redbook, Sports Illustrated for Kids,* and *Teen.*

Tobacco advertising in magazines clearly targets specific populations. The American Council on Science and Health studied tobacco advertising in women's magazines as well as the coverage of smoking and health issues. In their 2004 report, the ACSH found that tobacco advertising has declined but that less than 2 percent of magazine articles on health mention smoking or tobacco. Of the magazines surveyed, *Self, Prevention,* and *Woman's Day* published the most articles on smoking. There was a clear trend, with the publications with the most tobacco ads having the least coverage of smoking and health, and some, such as *Elle, Vogue,* and *Harper's Bazaar,* even sent positive messages about smoking to their readers.

A study of the advertising in men's and women's magazines as well as magazines in Spanish, conducted by San Diego State University, documented differences in both the number and type of ads in each of these publications. By comparing *Cosmopolitan* and *Glamour* to *Cosmopolitan en Español* and *Glamour en Español,* the authors could demonstrate that Latinas are targeted by far more ads for menthol cigarettes.

The same research team also showed menthol cigarettes were also more frequently marketed to African Americans. Menthol cigarettes are associated with a higher incidence of lung cancer, and lung malignancies occur more often in African Americans than in whites. In 2004, the R.J. Reynolds Tobacco Company settled a lawsuit with Illinois, Maryland, and New York over a promotion for *Kool* cigarettes that allegedly used hip-hop music to market the product to African American children. The company agreed to alter its practices and to pay $1.46 million towards youth smoking prevention.

The following list shows some major publications accepting tobacco ads likely to be read by minors, and magazines that have chosen not to accept this advertising. They are graded based on their ads and content, tobacco and lung cancer education, and potential impact.

A+ -Long standing policy of not accepting smoking ads

***Reader's Digest*:** Stopped accepting cigarette ads in 1924. Published an influential article, "Cancer by the Carton," in 1952.

***Good Housekeeping*:** In 1952, the Good Housekeeping Institute recognized the dangers of smoking, and the magazine stopped accepting tobacco ads.

B -Currently prints no tobacco advertising

Discover
Family Fun
Guitar Player
National Geographic
Ski Magazine
Skiing Magazine

LIMITED WARRANTY TO CONSUMERS
Good Housekeeping
Promises
REPLACEMENT OR REFUND IF DEFECTIVE

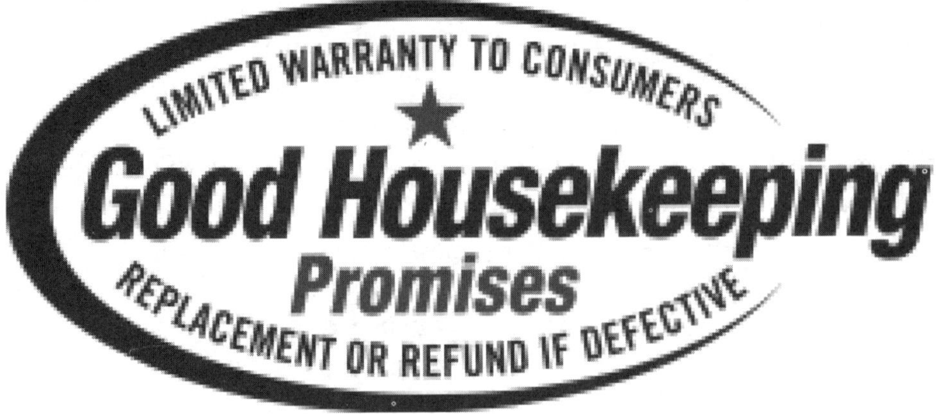

Figure 5.3 The famous Good Housekeeping Seal of Approval

Recent medical researches on the relationship of smoking and lung cancer

Cancer by the Carton

Figure 5.4 The title of the *Cancer by the Carton* article published in *Reader's Digest* December 1952.

D -Has tobacco advertising, but does have articles on smoking and health

Ladies Home Journal: Despite extensive pressure from readers, this widely read and influential magazine still accepts tobacco advertising. To their credit, they have cut back and have published articles on smoking, including a recent article on teenage tobacco addiction. But if *Good Housekeeping* wised up in 1952, what is taking *Ladies Home Journal* so long?

Newsweek: *Newsweek* has a circulation of over four million and a readership of twenty-one million, and it carries extensive tobacco advertising. They did print an article in April 2004 on smoking and lung cancer in women.

Time- Like *Newsweek,* this magazine brings tobacco advertising into millions of homes.

F -Tobacco ads and no coverage on tobacco and health

People, People En Español: This widely read magazine accepts tobacco advertising and has virtually no coverage of the effects of smoking on **people**.

Sports Illustrated: This magazine has a wide youth readership, particularly among males.

Harpers' Bazaar: A fashion magazine read by many young girls and women, it often has multiple tobacco ads per issue.

Cosmopolitan: While most readers of *Cosmo* are young adult women, considerable numbers of female minors read this magazine. *Cosmopolitan* features heavy tobacco advertising and virtually no information on the health effects of tobacco.

Ebony: This highly influential publication is a major source of tobacco advertising that targets African Americans.

Maxxim: While the target audience of *Maxxim* is clearly adult males, millions of underage boys see it.

***Car and Driver, Esquire, Entertainment, Field and Stream, Fortune, GQ, Marie Claire, Road and Track, Essence, Glamour, Motor Trend, Outdoor Life, Parade, Vogue, Rolling Stone, Playboy,* and many others.**

Convenience stores and Gas stations

With laws banning tobacco ads on billboards, advertising at service stations, convenience stores, retail stores, and grocery stores has become a major source of cigarette marketing. Many of these stores receive money to carry tobacco ads and promotions and are the contact points for promotional campaigns. Minors are regularly exposed to this advertising, and many teens and minors buy their tobacco at convenience stores and gas stations. Children readily detect hypocrisy. Being told not to smoke yet seeing tobacco ads, cigarettes for sale, and adults smoking can only cause confusion and increase their curiosity.

The National Association of Convenience Stores (NACS) stated that in 2005 there were 140,655 convenience stores in the United States, and that in 2003 the sale of cigarettes and other tobacco products made up over 34 percent of the in-store sales at these stores. Tobacco accounts for more sales at these stores than food, drinks, candy, snacks, and milk combined. In total, tobacco brings in a whopping $46 billion in revenue and $8.9 billion in profits. According to the Management Science Associates data, the convenience store industry's share of the cigarette market grew to 62 percent in 2003.

Needless to say, the convenience store lobby wants to protect their tobacco cash cow. "The NACS strongly opposes any effort to increase the federal excise tax on tobacco," says their web site. They also oppose granting the FDA the authority to regulate the sale of tobacco. "NACS opposes the federal regulation over the retail sale of tobacco products. NACS has long advocated that the sale of tobacco be regulated at the state, rather than federal, level where regulation is most effective." While every state has laws outlawing tobacco sales to minors and regulating the industry, the laws are unevenly enforced, and largely ineffective.

Not all service stations and convenience stores have the same involvement in advertising. Many convenience stores and service stations are independently owned, and so policies change from region to region. A large consumer movement to reduce tobacco advertising could be effective at eliminating advertising in store windows and on the property. Companies are highly tuned to customer demand. All major hotels have nonsmoking rooms and floors and several have gone completely smoke-free. Restaurants, airlines, and car rental companies have implemented similar policies. We now fully recognize the health effects of secondhand smoke and work to protect nonsmokers. A similar recognition of the health consequences of tobacco advertising on children could lead to voluntary actions by companies selling or marketing tobacco products.

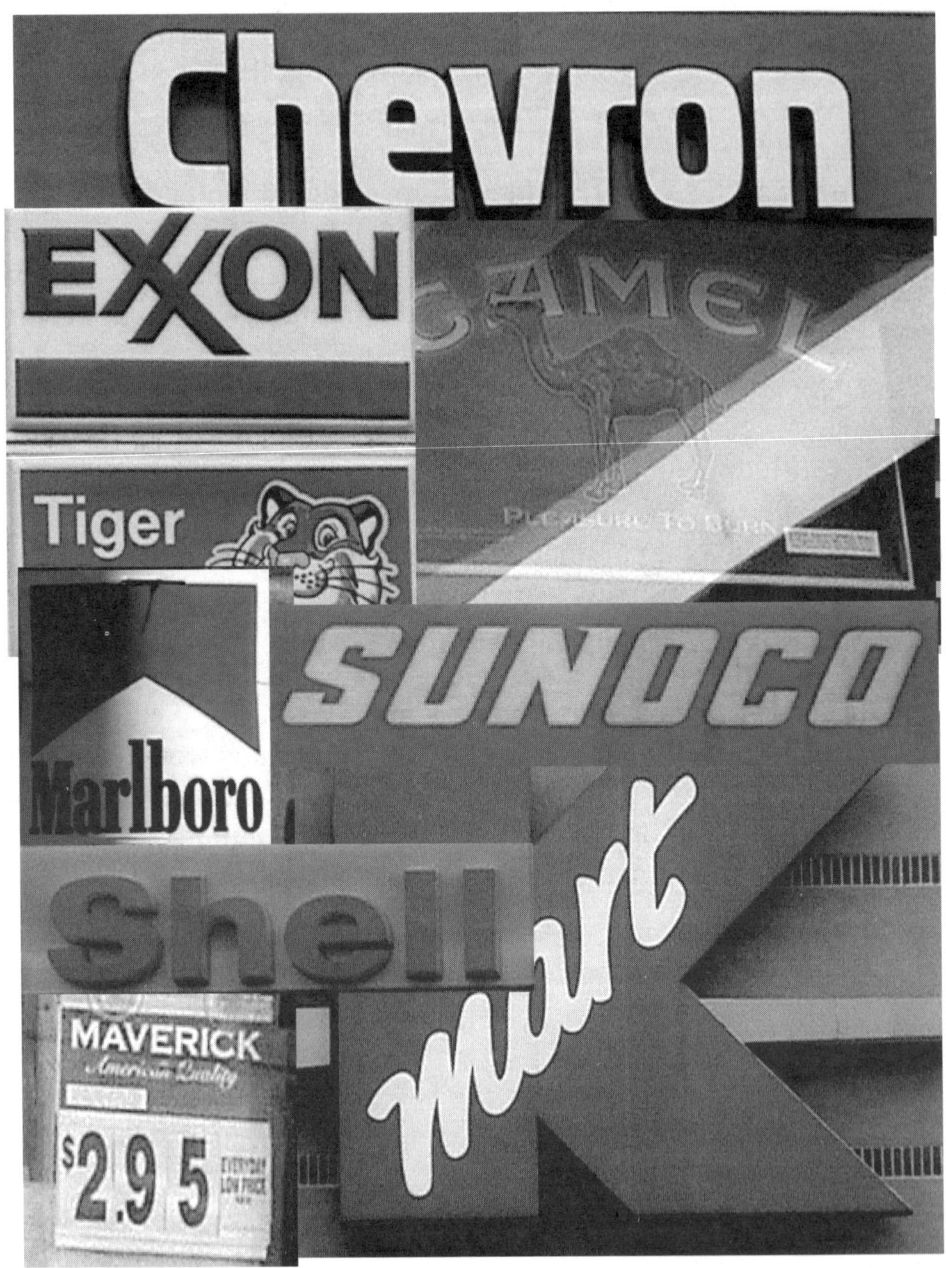

Figure 5.5 Collage of Cigarette retailers and ads.

What can you do?

- Become educated and involved in tobacco exposure, advertising, and sale issues.

- Watch for evidence of tobacco use by your children, and make sure tobacco in your home is not available to youngsters.

- Subscribe to tobacco-free publications.

- Write and email your favorite magazines to reduce or eliminate tobacco ads and support this effort.

- Urge your local convenience store and service station to reduce advertising or eliminate sales.

- Shop at stores with a policy of not selling tobacco products, and talk to the owners that do and tell them of your views.

- Write to companies who are major retailers and advertisers of tobacco and encourage them to reconsider their policies.

Chapter 6. The States and Smoking

How Does Your State Measure Up?

The United States has always been known for the unique character of each of its fifty states. Americans have long fought for the rights of individual communities to control their lives. The history of tobacco cultivation, smoking and government regulation is very different from one state to another. Tobacco is a major crop for several states. Over 435 thousand tons of tobacco is grown each year in the United States, with most of coming from six Southern states. Many powerful Senators and Representatives come from these states and have had a great influence on tobacco legislation.

One example of the influence of tobacco states has been the regulation of nicotine as a drug. Up until 1906 the United States had an essentially unregulated drug system. Virtually anyone could sell drugs and preparations such as "patent medicines." Even opiates like morphine and cocaine were legal. The Pure Food and Drug Act of 1906 and the revised version of 1938 created government regulation

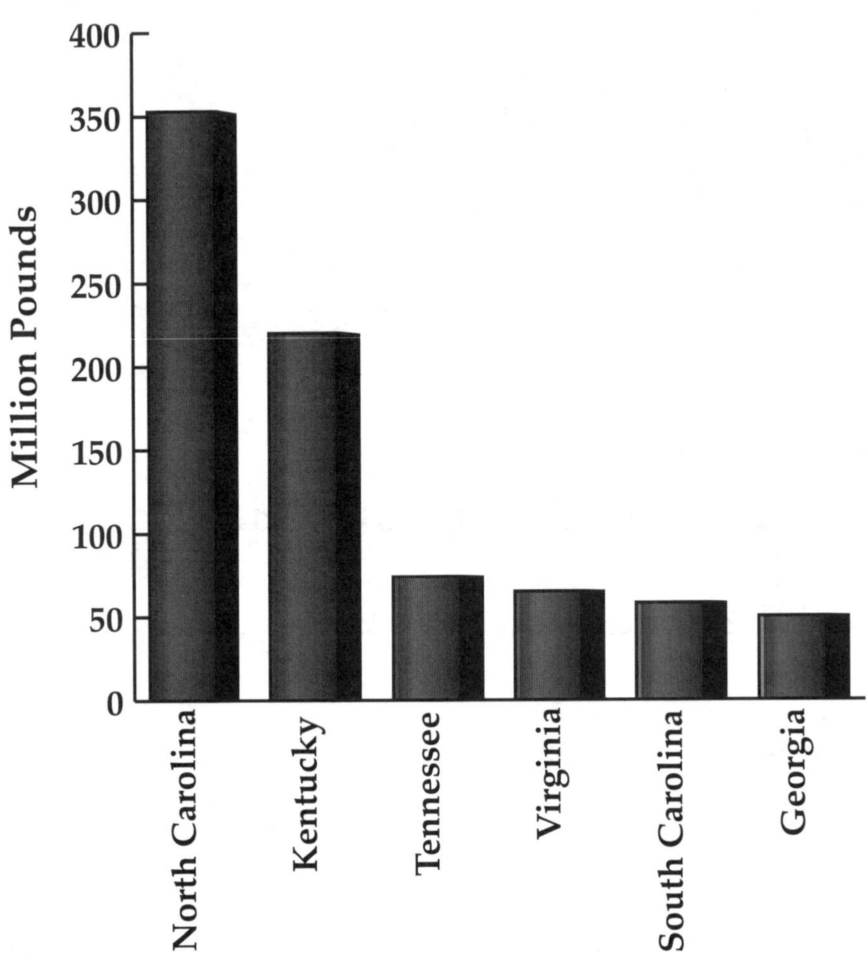

Figure 6.1 Major Tobacco Producing States. The tobacco production in millions of pounds is shown for the top six states. All other states produce less than 11,000,000 pounds (From the USDA, National Agriculture Statistics Service).

of pharmaceuticals, food additives, and health care devices. However, in drafting the food and drug legislation, the Southern states had tobacco products excluded from the law. To this date, despite the fact that cigarettes are a highly engineered and processed delivery device for the drug nicotine, tobacco products are unregulated. Other nicotine delivery products such as gum and patches, however, are regulated. In 1996, the FDA passed a rule restricting the sale and distribution of cigarettes and smokeless tobacco products to children and adolescents. The FDA also ruled that cigarettes and smokeless tobacco products are combination products consisting of a drug (nicotine) and device components intended to deliver nicotine to the body.

However, the FDA's rule was challenged by the tobacco industry and in 2000 the Supreme Court ruled in a five to four decision that the FDA has no authority to regulate tobacco. Legislation has been filed in Congress to grant the FDA such authority but the bills have never passed. Interestingly, the Philip Morris Company now favors FDA regulation of tobacco, whereas the other tobacco companies do not. Philip Morris sells more cigarettes than all other companies combined, and experts believe that FDA regulation could drive the smaller companies out of business leaving Philip Morris in an even better financial position.

The growth of tobacco plants has been highly regulated since the Great Depression. Government price supports and crop insurance were put in place to protect the income of farmers. In addition, a quota system has restricted the amount of tobacco that can be grown, and thereby keeping the price high. Tobacco can only be planted if the grower owns or rents a tobacco quota. This quota system is being phased out with a $10 billion dollar buyout program over the next several years. Once this program ends, tobacco can be grown anywhere, and prices may decline substantially.

Tobacco Addiction

The key to reducing smoking is to cut down on addiction in the young smoker. The rate of smoking varies dramatically from state to state. One state has by far the lowest rate of tobacco use for both underage children (7 percent) and adults (13 percent). It is not the state with the highest tax, nor does it spend the most on tobacco education. This interesting state is also not a 'liberal' state with extensive anti-smoking legislation. But as soon as you read the name of the state you will know why.

Did you guess it? The state with the lowest tobacco use, by far, is Utah. Ah ha, you now say! Of course. Utah is the state where over one half of its citizens belong to the Church of Jesus Christ of the Latter Day Saints (Mormons). In the Mormon faith, the members are instructed to avoid the use of tobacco. Consequently, most children in Mormon families do not see adults smoking or have access to tobacco. In fact, children in all nonsmoking households have a two to three fold lower rate of smoking. This observation confirms that the influence of family is one of the strongest forces in determining whether a child will smoke or not.

The remaining states have underage smoking rates as high as 36 percent in South Carolina and as low as 14 percent in Idaho. In general the states that grow most of the country's tobacco have the highest rates of smoking. These states also tend to have the lowest taxes on tobacco, and they spend little on tobacco cessation and education. The exceptions are Virginia and Georgia where underage smoking is relatively low and spending on tobacco education is greater.

Childhood Smoking Rates

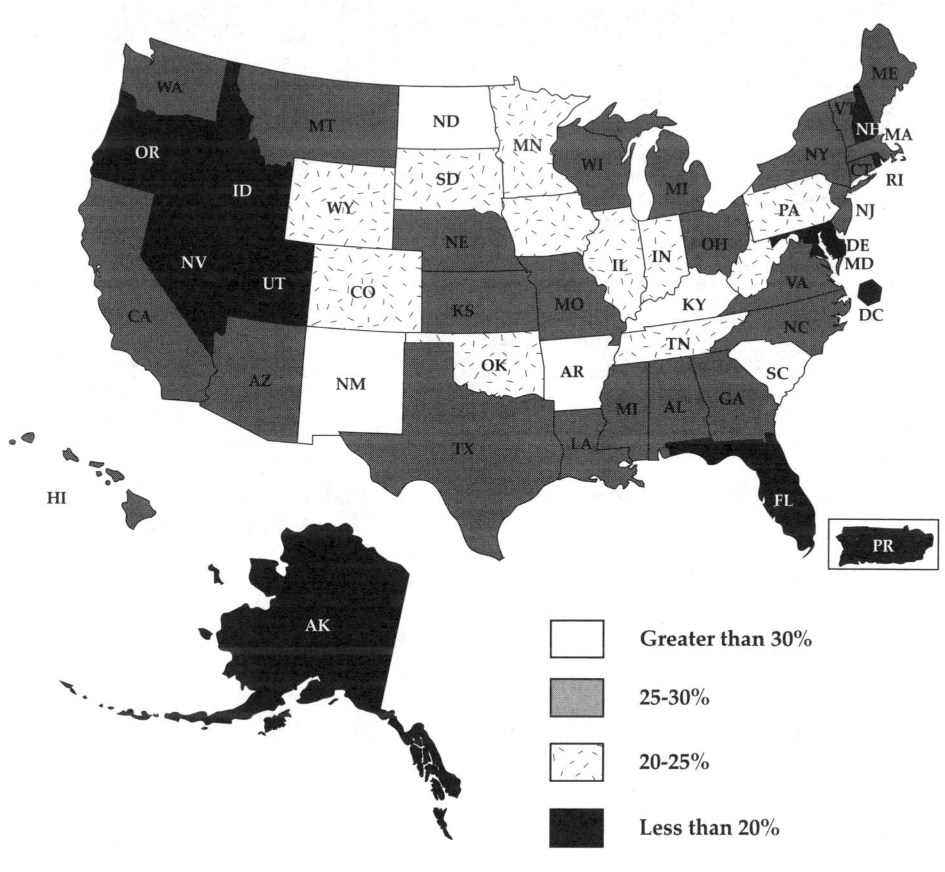

Figure 6.2 Map of childhood smoking rates. The rate of underage smoking in each state is shown.

Ranking of the Big 6 Tobacco Producing States

State	Tobacco Production	Teen Smoking	Adult Smoking	Tax
North Carolina	1	32	41	50
Kentucky	2	48	51	51
Tennessee	3	41	48	44
Virginia	4	16	36	44
South Carolina	5	50	44	49
Georgia	6	13	28	39

The states that grow the most tobacco are ranked in comparison to the other states and Washington, D.C., in their rate of teen and adult smoking, tax on tobacco and spending on tobacco cessation and education. For teen and adult smoking, 1 is the state with the lowest rate and 51 the highest. For Tax, 1 is the state with the highest tax or spending, 51 the lowest.

Taxing and Spending

There is an old saying in government that "if you want less of something, tax it." Many states apply this philosophy to tobacco products, and cigarettes have at least some level of tax in all of the states, from seven cents per pack in South Carolina to $2.40 per pack in Rhode Island. Many studies show that raising the taxes on cigarettes lowers consumption. When the cost goes up, some people smoke less or quit, and price is a barrier keeping some young people from starting. According to TobaccoFreeKids.org, "[E]xperience in state after state show[s] that higher cigarette taxes are one of the most effective ways to reduce smoking among both youth and adults. Every 10 percent increase in the price of cigarettes will reduce youth smoking by about 7 percent and overall cigarette consumption by about 4 percent."

The difference in the price of cigarettes from one region to another can lead to problems such as smuggling. The most extreme example occurred in Canada, where, in the 1980s, the government dramatically increased the tax on cigarettes, making them more expensive than in the United States. Canadian cigarettes exported to the United States were often smuggled back into Canada. A large organized criminal operation developed to bring cheaper cigarettes from the United States into Canada, leading to a great increase in crime. At the height of the smuggling, contraband cigarettes were estimated to constitute 60 percent of the market. In 1994, the tax was reduced, and the crime spree subsided.

In the United States, most high-tax states allow only one to two cartons of cigarettes at a time to be brought into the state. Both small-scale and large-scale smuggling occurs between low-tax and high-tax states, and this business is estimated to be worth over $1 billion per year for the smugglers. The illegal cigarette trade includes the transport of cigarettes from low-tax to high-tax states as well as the smuggling of counterfeit smokes into the country. A large underground cigarette market encourages underage smokers, who obtain tobacco outside of traditional channels.

Cigarette taxes have been criticized for being regressive. That means they are particularly hard on poor people and people with a fixed income. If a person without much money has to spend more on cigarettes, they have less to spend on food, clothes, and other necessities. The hope, of course, is that these individuals will smoke less or quit, but many do not. Obviously, taxation should be followed up with smoking cessation and education programs.

Tobacco taxes fall into a group, including taxes on alcohol and gambling referred to as 'sin taxes.' Sin taxes represent a government attempt to restrict otherwise legal behaviors by making them more expensive in an effort to generate money for the government to combat the effects of the sin on society. Some communities have even extended this concept to the taxation of fast food and junk food. On the one side, it is argued that the government has to pay for the health consequences of smoking, drinking, gambling, and poor eating habits through the treatment of cancer, heart disease, and other social problems. Therefore, it is argued, the government should collect money from these individuals to help pay for the expenses which result from their need for medical care for smoking-related diseases. On the other hand, sin taxes have been criticized as being misguided. For the government to profit from the 'sin' would bring about a conflict of interest situation. If sin taxes reach high levels, people will find underground sources of the product to avoid the government tax.

Many studies demonstrate that the cost of cigarettes has an effect on underage smoking. The more expensive cigarettes are, the lower the rate of teen smoking. Preventing children from smoking in the beginning is the most effective way to reduce tobacco-related disease. Therefore, increasing tobacco taxation across the states at a moderate level and using the money to increase education, smoking cessation programs, and to reduce underage sales represents progressive government policy.

Smoking Cessation

The Centers for Disease Control has set a goal for each state to spend about $6 per person on smoking education and cessation programs. Currently, only four states spend at this level, and many states use most or all of their tobacco settlement and excise tax revenue elsewhere. A few states have initiated extensive campaigns to reduce smoking and have seen dramatic results in limiting underage smoking and tobacco-related deaths. The state of Vermont carried out a campaign from 1985-1989 judged to be the most effective for each dollar spent. The campaign featured youthful actors, stressed the advantages of nonsmoking, and provided tips on skills for refusing tobacco. A successful California program started in 1990 focused on the deceptive advertising of the tobacco industry and the adverse health effects of secondhand smoke. Massachusetts, Florida, and Minnesota carried out effective campaigns that reduced youth smoking rates. The most useful ingredients in these campaigns are clear, consistent messages and the use of young spokespeople to deliver them. Several states (Michigan, Washington D.C., New Hampshire, South Dakota, Missouri, and Tennessee) do not spend any of the settlement funds on smoking cessation programs. Only Maine, Colorado, Delaware, Mississippi, and Arkansas spend at least the amount recommended by the CDC.

Smoking at Work

A considerable amount of smoking takes place in social settings since smoking was once considered an acceptable social activity. A number of businesses allow smoking by their customers, particularly bars, restaurants, and casinos. However, smoking patrons create health problems for the employees and the customers. In 1988, smoking was banned on all domestic airline flights of less than two hours and, in 1990, on all flights of six hours of less. Today, virtually all commercial airline flights are smoke-free, as are most airports, leading to improved health for pilots, flight attendants, and travelers. Efforts are being made at the city and state level to ban smoking in all workplaces. As of 2006, fourteen states have passed legislation banning or restricting smoking at work. In addition, numerous counties and cities have passed similar bans, and citizens groups in most of the remaining states are fighting for similar legislation. One of the consistent objections to such bans is that it will hurt business at bars and restaurants. However, studies consistently show that business increases following these bans. In Rhode Island, in the six months after the smoke-free law first took effect, sales tax collections on meals and beverages rose 8.2 percent over the same period in the prior year.

"All workers (including office, restaurant, bar, bingo, bowling, casino, tavern, pub, and nightclub workers) deserve a safe, healthy, smoke-free work environment," says Joe Cherner, founder of BREATHE — Bar and Restaurant Employees Advocating Together for a Healthy Environment. "Laws should treat the health of all workers equally. Bar and restaurant workers should have the same right to a smoke-free work environment as everyone else. No worker should have to breathe tobacco smoke pollution to hold a job, because it causes cancer, respiratory illness, and heart disease."

At the Federal level, in 2004, the Secretary of the Department of Health and Human Services (HHS), Tommy Thompson, ordered that all HHS facilities become tobacco-free. He also ordered that free smoking cessation assistance be given to any employee requesting it. The tobacco ban was part of a program to encourage Americans to quit and included a new hotline (1-800-QUIT-NOW) and a web site (www.smokefree.gov) offering online advice and downloadable information to make quitting easier. "What starts as a single puff can become a death sentence for millions of Americans," said Secretary Thompson. "Americans want to quit smoking, and they should quit smoking. These initiatives will help Americans kick the habit and save their own lives."

At one Health and Human Services location, the National Cancer Institute facility in Frederick, Maryland; fifty employees took advantage of the opportunity to quit. This shows that even at an institution dedicated to cancer research many employees smoke. They can be convinced to quit by banning smoking in the workplace and providing them with help to quit.

Internationally, smoking bans in the workplace are being passed at a rapid pace. Nine of the thirteen provinces in Canada have banned workplace smoking, as have the countries of Bermuda, Bhutan, England, Ireland, Italy, Malta, New Zealand, Norway, Scotland, Spain, Sweden, Uganda, Uruguay, and Wales.

Studies in Italy, published in the medical journal *Annals of Oncology,* show that after the ban in workplaces was passed, the consumption of cigarettes declined. "The results of our study on the first extensive smoking ban in a large country show the advantages of smoke-free legislation, which may have major public health implications," wrote the authors. The largest declines in smoking were seen in young people (23 percent for the fifteen to twenty-four -year-old age group) and among women (a fall of 11 percent). Over

90 percent of the public supports the ban and business has increased in Italian bars and restaurants. Polls taken in many countries and communities show that 70 to 80 percent of the public favors banning smoking in workplaces.

One of the groups most in favor of eliminating smoking in bars and clubs are musicians. Musicians often play in smoke-filled rooms, and the constant exposure to smoke is a major health hazard. Priscilla Giles, secretary and treasurer of the New Hampshire chapter of the American Federation of Musicians, said her members cannot simply change jobs. She said no other workers are expected to make those kinds of choices, and "you shouldn't expect someone to find a new job because they don't want to breathe a hazardous substance."

At my scientific research laboratory, we work with a number of hazardous chemicals and radioactive compounds. If a woman tells her supervisor that she is pregnant, she must be given a workplace that is as free as possible from anything that might be hazardous to her unborn child. Why are we excluding tobacco, one of the most hazardous of compounds, from similar restrictions?

States and Medical Coverage

One of the most cost effective ways that states can reduce smoking and its ill effects is by providing for medical coverage for smoking cessation. While most medical insurance companies cover the costs of smoking cessation treatments, many people lack medical insurance. One of the national health objectives set by the Centers for Disease Control for 2010 is to provide coverage by Medicaid in the fifty states and the District of Columbia (DC) for nicotine-dependence treatment. Surprisingly, only thirty-nine states offer any coverage for Medicare patients, and four of these cover only pregnant women. Only New Jersey and Oregon provide coverage for all of the recommended drug therapies and counseling programs recommended by the CDC. Individuals on Medicare have a 50 percent higher rate of smoking than the general population, so these smokers are a particularly attractive group to target.

The States in Court

Despite the imperfect record of many states on smoking issues, it is the Attorney Generals of the states that have taken the lead in the courts. Large lawsuits, initially brought by individual states resulted in the massive out-of-court settlement in 1998 with forty-six of the states, resulting in the payment of more than $200 billion over twenty-five years in exchange for marketing restrictions, including the elimination of cartoon characters and outdoor advertising.

Individual states' Attorney Generals have also forced policy changes by companies marketing tobacco. Threats of lawsuits led to the introduction of the *We Card* program, providing voluntary compliance by many retailers, including training of salespeople and the requirement for identification by purchasers that appear to be under twenty-seven years of age. Individual and group lawsuits have been brought against numerous retailers, such as 7-Eleven, Safeway, and CVS, following repeated violations of selling to minors, self-service cigarette displays, and outdoor signs near schools. In 2006, CVS, the second largest drugstore chain, paid a $250,000 fine to forty states and agreed to undertake more stringent training of their sales force and better compliance with the law.

Grading the States

To determine how each state is performing in combating tobacco addictions, a grading system was created. The policies and smoking rates of each state in four categories (taxes, spending on smoking cessation, and teen and adult smoking rates) was used to generate a ranking for each state. A grade of A was given to the states doing the best job, and the worst states received an F.

This grading system allows one to readily compare the commitment of individual states. Through citizen pressure, your state government can be made to do more to fight tobacco addiction. Consumers could choose where to spend their vacation dollars based on this information.

Grading the States on Smoking Rates, Tobacco Taxes, and Prevention

A

Utah*
Maryland
Washington*
California*
Vermont*
Hawaii
New York*
Maine*
Rhode Island*
Massachusetts*
Arizona
Puerto Rico

B

New Jersey*
Connecticut*
Idaho*
Washington D.C.*
Oregon
Montana*
Alaska
Pennsylvania
Nevada
Delaware*

C

Kansas
Wisconsin
New Mexico
Ohio
Minnesota
Florida*
Georgia
Virginia
Wyoming

D

Michigan
Nebraska
New Hampshire
Illinois
North Dakota
Colorado
Arkansas
Louisiana
Texas
Mississippi

F

Iowa
Kentucky
North Carolina
Missouri
West Virginia

South Dakota
Tennessee
South Carolina
Oklahoma
Indiana
Alabama

* States with smoking bans

What can you do?

- **Write to your state government to urge them to do more to prevent teen smoking and provide education.**

- **Choose to vacation in those states with the most proactive smoking policies.**

- **Are you involved in planning a company meeting or convention? Pick a city in a state with progressive tobacco policies (for example Salt Lake City, New York, Seattle, Honolulu, Boston, Baltimore, Providence, Portland, ME, Los Angeles, San Francisco, or Phoenix).**

Chapter 7 From Farm to Finger

Cigarette Companies from Amoco to Wal-Mart

For thousands of years, Native Americans cultivated the tobacco plant — selecting ever-potent strains, harvesting and drying the leaves, and smoking them. The practice is believed to have developed among the civilizations of South America as early as 3000 to 5000 B.C. By the time Europeans arrived in the Americas, tobacco use was found throughout North and South America. When the plant was first presented to Columbus, he saw no use for the smelly stuff and tossed it into the sea. But his sailors and other explorers brought the plant back to Europe, and from there it was introduced to Asia and the rest of the world. Smoking and medicinal uses of tobacco became popular, and tobacco cultivation in the New World began in earnest in the 1500s. Because tobacco leaves can be dried and stored for a long time and are valuable, tobacco became a form of currency.

The use of tobacco as money would last into the 1800s, and Thomas Jefferson's grade school tuition was paid in tobacco.

In these early years, tobacco use was largely confined to the smoking of pipes and cigars, and chewing tobacco. The use of snuff became popular in the 1700s, and Napoleon used seven pounds per month. The first cigarettes were created and smoked by Europeans in Spain in the 1600s. Cigarettes gained in popularity in both Europe and the United States in the 1800s, and the first American cigarette factories were established in the 1850s. However, it was the invention of a cigarette-rolling machine that led to an explosion of production and a shift in tobacco use. James Buchanan "Buck" Duke bought the first such machines and built a tobacco empire. Duke's American Tobacco Company came to control 90 percent of the world's tobacco market. But, in 1911, the company was broken up as a monopoly. One year before his death, Duke founded his now famous university.

Today's tobacco market is far different than it was in colonial days. Although the plant is still grown on many farms, most of the leaves are purchased and distributed by a few multinational corporations and sold to the large cigarette producers. Many corporations make at least some of their money in the production, distribution, marketing, and sale of tobacco products. One way for the concerned consumer and citizen to fight back against the damage caused to children by this industry is to avoid buying the products of tobacco-associated companies and to limit investment in these firms. Until now, there has not been a comprehensive list of such firms. This chapter provides a description of those companies and their products.

Major Tobacco Companies

Tobacco products are produced by a small number of multinational corporations. These companies often own other businesses. Most tobacco companies are publicly traded on the stock market and make up significant portions of many investment portfolios. The largest producer of cigarettes in the United States is

Philip Morris, a division of the **Altria Group** (Stock symbol **MO**). Philip Morris sold 187 billion cigarettes in the United States in 2004, which represents about half of the total cigarettes sold in the country. Altria/Philip Morris sells about 15 percent of the cigarettes sold worldwide (they produced 761 billion of the 5.1 **trillion** cigarettes sold in the world in 2004) and they have 15 percent or more of the market in over seventy different countries. These sales resulted in $17.5 billion in revenue in 2004 for domestic sales and $39.5 billion in international sales. Altria also owns **Kraft Foods,** the distributor of such products as Post cereals, Jell-O, Maxwell House coffee, Grape-Nuts, Cream of Wheat, and Velveeta cheese.

R.J. Reynolds (**RAI**) is the second-largest cigarette producer in the country, and they merged United States business operations with Brown and Williamson Tobacco, owned by the **British American Tobacco Company**. The merged R.J. Reynolds produces about 31 percent of the cigarettes sold in the United States, a total of ninety-four billion. The holding company **Loews Corporation** owns the **Carolina Group** (**CG**), the owner of Lorillard Tobacco, the oldest tobacco company in the country. Loews also owns Loews hotels, CNA insurance, and Bulova watches. Lorillard accounts for about 9 percent of cigarettes sold in the United States. The **US Smokeless Tobacco Corp.** (**UST**) is the primary producer of smokeless tobacco in the United States. UST's most popular smokeless tobacco products account for over $2 billion in sales per year. These four companies produce the vast majority of tobacco products manufactured and marketed in our country. Reducing or eliminating your investment in these companies sends a message that you do not support their products, or their behavior. Here is a list of the major tobacco companies and their stock symbols.

Stock Symbols for Tobacco Companies

Symbol	Company Name
MO	Altria/Philip Morris
RAI	R.J. Reynolds
CG	Loews Carolina Group
UST	US Smokeless Tobacco Co.

While you might not hold individual shares in a tobacco company, 30 to 40 percent of mutual funds invest significant amounts in these corporations. Here is a list of the ten most widely held Mutual Funds and their investment in tobacco companies. Funds that have no individual tobacco company making up more than 1 percent of their holdings, and no holdings in companies profiting from cigarettes, are given a grade of A; funds with only "other tobacco" get a grade of B, or C; and funds with major tobacco holdings, D or F.

Top Mutual Funds and Tobacco Holdings

Symbol	Fund	Tobacco Holdings	Grade
VFINX	Vanguard 500 Index	Altria 1.05%	C
FMAGX	Fidelity Magellan	**NONE**	**A**
AIVSX	American Funds Invmt Co of Amer A	Altria 4.71%	
AWSHX	American Funds Washington Mutual A	Altria 4.56%	F
AGTHX	American Funds Washington Mutual A	Altria 1.92%	D
FCNTX	Fidelity Contrafund	**NONE**	**A**
DODGX	Dodge & Cox Stock	**NONE**	**A**
AMECX	American Funds Inc Fund of Amer A	Altria 1.92%	D
AEPGX	American Funds EuroPacific Gr A	**NONE**	**A**
FLPSX	Fidelity Low-Priced Stock	**NONE**	**A**

Other tobacco companies

In addition to the cigarette manufacturers, many companies are involved in the growth of tobacco, distribution of cigarettes, and the advertisement and sale of cigarettes. Major growers and producers include **Alliance One International** (**AOI**), a company resulting from the merger of **Dimon, Incorporated** (**DMN**), and **Standard Commercial Corp.** (**STW**). **Universal Corp.** (**UVV**) owns the Universal Leaf Tobacco Company, a leaf tobacco merchant. **Vector Group, Ltd.** (**VGR**) sells cigarettes in the United States through Liggett Group, Inc. **Star Scientific, Inc.** (**STSI**) manufactures and sells discount cigarettes. **Wellstone Filters, Inc.** (**WFLT.OB**) is involved in research, development, and marketing for the tobacco industry, as well as in cigarette distribution.

Cigarette Distribution, Marketing, and Sales

Cigarettes are sold throughout the country in thousands of stores. They include grocery stores and large retailers, drug stores, liquor and tobacco stores, convenience stores, and gas stations. Therefore, there are many companies profiting from these sales. While many regional grocery and convenience store chains are privately owned, the national chains are publicly traded on the stock markets. The largest cigarette retailer in the United States is **Wal-Mart (WMT)**. Other major cigarette retailers include **7-Eleven** (**SE**), **Sears Holding Company (SHLD)** through its subsidiary Kmart, **Kroger Co. (KR), Albertson's, Inc. (ABS), Safeway, Inc. (SWY), Shell (RDS), Exxon Mobil Corp. (XOM), British Petroleum/Amoco PLC (BP), ChevronTexaco Corp. (CVX), Rite Aid Corp. (RAD), CVS Corp. (CVS),** and **Walgreen Co. (WAG).** The major distributor of cigarettes is McLane Company, Inc., a wholly owned subsidiary of **Berkshire Hathaway, Inc. (BRK-A).**

Many of these companies have signed on to the *We Card* program, to avoid legal action from the state Attorney Generals. This program provides training for retailers and their employees on preventing underage sales. Although sales to minors have been reduced in some regions, children are able to buy cigarettes at these stores 20 to 40 percent of the time. A recent compliance check by the police in Frederick, Maryland cited eighteen out of twenty-five stores for selling tobacco to minors. Maryland has now implemented a tougher law providing stiffer fines and suspensions for repeat offenders. The compliance checks found that the larger stores, including Wal-Mart, were the worst offenders. The state of California sued the Safeway Corporation for failing to adequately halt tobacco sales to minors, but in most states, compliance enforcement is minimal.

As discussed in Chapter 5, a large number of magazines and newspapers advertise tobacco products. Private companies produce many of these publications. However two corporations stand out as major tobacco advertisers. The **Time Warner (TWX)**/AOL corporation publishes *Time* magazine and many other magazines with cigarette ads. The **Washington Post Co.** (**WPO**) owns *Newsweek* magazine. *Time* and *Newsweek* are noteworthy because they are sent to millions of homes and to schools. Although many schools remove tobacco ads from their magazines, not all do. In addition, as important news magazines, there is at least an appearance of conflict of interest, and studies have found publications with tobacco advertising do not produce as many articles on the health effects of smoking as do similar magazines without such ads.

The Media

Smoking is actively depicted in a large number of films and television programs. The Centers for Disease Control consistently names the depiction of smoking in the media by popular actors (and cartoon characters) as a major influence in the choice of children to smoke. Scientific studies, in medical journals such as *The Lancet,* document an association between frequent exposures to smoking in movies with a higher risk of smoking in ten- to fourteen-year-olds. Smoking amongst children could be cut in half if children's exposure to smoking in the media could be eliminated. In the past, the tobacco companies are known to have directly and indirectly paid movie studios, directors, and actors to place their products in films. The studios and the tobacco companies claim that the payments have stopped, but smoking depictions and product placements continue to show up in movies including those rated PG and PG-13 and in movies targeted towards youths.

Dr. Stanton A. Glantz, professor of medicine at the University of California, San Francisco, has created the Smoke Free Movies project to publicize the depiction of smoking in films and change this practice (http://smokefreemovies.ucsf.edu). The group proposes giving movies with smoking characters an R rating unless the character is an actual historical figure or the adverse effects of smoking are clearly depicted. Smoke Free Movies also tracks movies with tobacco use. The companies most often displaying smoking are the **Sony Corp. (SNE)**, **The Walt Disney Co.** (**DIS**), and **Time Warner** (**TWX**). These three companies account for 60 percent of all smoking scenes in movies. Other major players include **Viacom, Inc. (VIA** and **VIA-B), General Electric Co. (GE)** (through ownership of Universal Studios) and **News Corporation. (NWS)** (owners of 20th Century Fox and Fox Studios). Tobacco use can also be seen on television, both on the networks (in Prime Time) and cable. One of the most famous recent television series, HBO's *Sex in the City*, featured a glamorous, independent woman who regularly smoked. Not only is smoking shown on television and in the movies, but the largest tobacco manufacturer's products are clearly displayed in these films. Does HBO or the film companies receive money from Philip Morris for this 'advertising'? As they are privately held companies, we don't know, but it seems unlikely that they would provide such product placement for free.

Individuals concerned about the effect of smoking on children's health can choose not to invest in companies profiting from tobacco marketing and write to them to encourage them to reduce or stop the sale and advertising of tobacco products. As 80 percent of consumers are nonsmokers, companies taking a stand on this issue are likely to gain a competitive advantage. Some concerned groups of stockholders have begun drafting shareholder resolutions to encourage companies to reduce or eliminate their involvement in profiting from tobacco. Several companies have taken independent stands against tobacco. The **Target Corp. (TGT)** is the only major retailer that does not sell tobacco products. The **McDonald's Corporation** (**MCD**) was one of the first restaurant chains to go smoke-free.

What can you do?

- Reduce your purchase of products and services from companies profiting from cigarettes.
- Write to companies you think would be receptive to your input on the subject.
- Consider selling any stock you own in these companies or introducing a shareholder resolution to change their policies.
- Seek out grocery, drug, and convenience stores and gas stations that do not advertise or sell tobacco
- Talk to local storeowners about your concerns

Chapter 8 Moving Ahead

The Future of Smoking

"Total prohibition of smoking in the workplace strongly affects industry volume. Smokers facing these restrictions consume 11 to 15 percent less than average and quit at a rate that is 84 percent higher than average. Only 6.4 to 10.3 percent of smokers face total workplace prohibition but these restrictions are rapidly becoming more common."

— Philip Morris Inter-Office Communication, January 22, 1992

In the 1600s, King James I of England described smoking as a filthy habit and banned it from the palace, yet the practice took hold in England and the rest of Europe. Since then, governments and organizations have fought against smoking and sought to reduce or eliminate it. However, the grip of nicotine is very strong, and once a person starts using tobacco, they are likely to continue for many years or for the rest of their life. About 50 percent of smokers try to quit each year, but only a fraction succeed. Most smokers want to stop.

Recent years have seen a dramatic increase in local, grass roots efforts to reduce smoking. Labor unions have fought for smoke-free workplaces, and twelve States have now banned smoking on the job (California, Delaware, New York, Connecticut, Maine, Massachusetts, Rhode Island, Montana, Vermont, Utah, Washington, and New Jersey), as have Puerto Rico and Washington D.C. Smoking restrictions in the workplace have also been passed in Florida, Georgia, Idaho, New Jersey, and South Dakota. In addition, consumers are starting to exercise their voice. Starting with the Comfort Inn Midtown in New York City, several hotels have gone fully smoke-free and have seen an increase in business, with 90 to 100 percent occupancy rates in most months, and reduced insurance and cleaning costs. The trend has spread to hotels in over thirty-six states (http://smokinghurts.com/Smoke-FreeHotels.htm). In 2005, the Westin hotel chain banned smoking in all of their United States and Canadian properties, and in 2006 the Marriott chain did the same. Both companies cited overwhelming demand by guests for nonsmoking rooms, and reduced costs as factors in the decision to go smokefree. Other hotel chains are expected to follow. The demand is there for a smoke-free environment, and those businesses that recognize this trend will benefit.

Recently, legislation has been approved in Arkansas and Utah to ban smoking in cars where children are present. Similar bills have been considered in New Jersey, California, and other states, and bans of smoking in all cars have been proposed. In a state where smoking bans on some beaches and parks are already in effect, the city of Calabasas, California, has enacted a ban on all outdoor smoking. There is considerable disagreement, even within the tobacco control community, on where to draw the line on protecting public health. In the end, each individual community will decide how strictly the government should regulate tobacco use.

The elimination of child labor, implementation of childhood vaccines, and advances in consumer safety and household safety led to remarkable advances in reducing infant and childhood mortality and improving children's lives. The most dangerous product to babies and children in our society today is tobacco, and it is time to act. The information provided above is meant to be a resource for you to make your own consumer choices. If you are concerned about the effect of tobacco products on the health of unborn children and babies, there are many things you can do to change the situation. If you feel that local, state, and federal governments can do more, by all means let them know. You as an individual and a consumer can make a difference!

The Future of Quitting

The success rate of conventional smoking cessation therapies is rather poor. Studies of smokers given both antianxiety drugs and nicotine replacement therapy show a twelve-month success rate of 27 percent. Because of the relative ineffectiveness of standard smoking cessation therapies, researchers have explored other options. Telephone help lines (also known as 'quit lines') are increasingly used to assist smokers in quitting. A central number, 1-800-QUIT-NOW, connects people in all fifty states to the resources in their area. Many health insurance plans and employers also cover telephone counseling and the service is free in several states. Some of the advantages of telephone counseling are the one-on-one interaction, smokers ability to arrange the calls to fit their schedules, and the mostly anonymous nature of the service. Studies have shown that these factors lead more people to sign up and more smokers to complete the program and successfully quit. One of the largest companies providing telephone counseling for smokers is Free and Clear, Inc. It provides services for many states, employers, and health care plans. Free and Clear has participated in several scientific studies sponsored by the National Cancer Institute, the CDC, and the Robert Wood Johnson Foundation. These studies have demonstrated the effectiveness of telephone-based programs and have helped to improve the approach.

A more controversial approach to quitting is the use of low-nicotine cigarettes. Several cigarette companies conducted studies on cigarettes with reduced levels of nicotine in the 1980s. In these studies, smokers became very unhappy with their smokes. They did not satisfy! In fact, a number of smokers using low nicotine cigarettes quit entirely. Needless to say, the tobacco companies dropped these products like a hot potato — until recently.

After the success of many lawsuits against the tobacco companies, one company, Liggett Vector Brands (formerly Liggett and Myers, one of the oldest tobacco companies) began producing new cigarette products. One of these, Quest, is a line of reduced-nicotine and nicotine-free cigarettes. These reduced-nicotine cigarettes are being marketed as one method to reduce nicotine dependence. Reduced-nicotine cigarettes are not safer, but if the smoker eventually quits, he or she will enjoy the health benefits.

The reason that reduced-nicotine cigarettes are effective in some smokers is clear. Smoking involves a long-practiced group of behaviors. Nicotine addicts often smoke in social settings and carry out rituals involving the handling, smelling, and lighting of the cigarette. All of these behaviors are linked, in the smoker's brain, with pleasure (although the 'pleasure' is actually the relief of their withdrawal symptoms).

Some smokers find it hard to give up, all at once, both the cigarettes and the nicotine. With low-nicotine cigarettes, the smoker gradually is weaned from the nicotine, and once the cigarette no longer provides pleasure, he or she can give that up too. This is the opposite approach to nicotine replacement therapy, where the cigarettes are given up first and the nicotine later. Few scientific studies have been performed with this approach. However, a Liggett company press release states that 33 to 54 percent of smokers in a study at Duke University Medical Center quit using the nicotine-free

Quest cigarette. Bennett S. LeBow, Chairman and Chief Executive Officer of Vector Group, said, "We are extremely encouraged by these test results. Although more research is necessary, we believe these results show real promise for the Quest technology as a smoking cessation aid."

There is one long-standing smoking cessation method claiming to have a very high success rate. Allen Carr is a former smoker from England who came across a method of quitting that worked for him. Mr. Carr is not a doctor nor a scientist, but he published a book on his method, entitled *The Easy Way to Stop Smoking*. This book is one of the best-selling tobacco-quitting self-help books in over twenty years and has been translated into twenty languages. Mr. Carr created a web-based program and a series of smoking cessation clinics, both of which claim a success rate of over 90 percent and offer a money-back guarantee.

How does the Easy Way method work? The book takes the reader through the reasons why smokers say they smoke and explains why so many methods fail. In addition, all the advantages of the nonsmoker are presented. The key to the Carr method is eliminating the idea that there is any positive aspect to smoking. Cigarettes do not taste good, relieve stress, improve concentration, or promote weight loss. Once the smoker comes to the conclusion that there is no benefit, he or she can willingly give them up, tackle the usually minor discomfort of nicotine withdrawal for a few weeks, and join the ranks of the nonsmoker.

Another innovative approach uses a small handheld computer called QuitKey. The smoker uses this device to track their tobacco use and to gradually reduce smoking. The addict smokes at their normal rate for the first seven days, recording into the device each cigarette smoked. From this information, the device learns the person's smoking pattern. Then the device develops a smoking cessation program, prompting the individual when to smoke the next cigarette. Withdrawal is accomplished gradually, and short-term setbacks can be accommodated and the smoker led back on track. The device was developed using government funding and has shown very promising success with a number of smokers.

There are also advances in pharmaceuticals to aid in quitting. The FDA has recently approved a new drug, Chantix™ (varenicline), from Pfizer, Inc. It is believed that Chantix acts by binding to some of the same receptors in the brain as nicotine, but Chantix appears to activate the receptors to a much lesser extent. If a person does smoke while taking Chantix, the drug may block nicotine from binding and lessen its' effects. The smoker needs to take Chantix two times per day for the duration of the treatment.

"Quitting smoking is challenging physiologically and psychologically," said Karen Katen, Pfizer vice chairman and president of Pfizer Human Health. "Oftentimes, smokers are very much on their own during the difficult quitting process. By developing Chantix to help people quit smoking, we hope to take a positive step toward improving the health of smokers, their families and friends, and society in general." For example, less than 7 percent of smokers who try to quit by themselves achieve at least one year of abstinence.

In two identically designed clinical studies approximately 44 percent of smokers taking Chantix quit smoking by the end of the twelve week treatment period, compared to approximately 30 percent taking Zyban and 18 percent who used a placebo (sugar pill). Pfizer is working with medical insurance companies to have the cost of the drug covered, and is also establishing the Get Quit™ Support Plan, a behavioral modification program offered at no additional cost to Chantix users, and is working with quitlines to help properly counsel Chantix users. Chantix has not been tested in pregnant or nursing women and is not prescribed for them at this point.

Another approach under development to help smokers quit is nicotine vaccines. These treatments would remove any nicotine from the bloodstream and block it from reaching the brain. After treatment with a vaccine, a person with a nicotine addiction could smoke or chew tobacco and not receive any of the nicotine. The vaccine typically kicks in gradually, lessening the withdrawal symptoms. A Florida biotech company, Nabi Biopharmaceuticals, has a nicotine vaccine called NicVAX showing promise in clinical studies. If the remaining studies are successful, the vaccine could be approved for doctors to prescribe in 2007.

In the end, the method of quitting is not critical. The important thing is to quit. Since most smokers want to quit, they should be offered as many options as possible and given adequate support. No one approach to giving up cigarettes will work for all smokers, so the best advice is to keep trying different strategies until you succeed.

CDC-Recommended Therapies

Therapy Type	Therapy
Drug Therapies	Nicotine Nasal Spray
	Nicotine Inhaler
	Nicotine Patch
	Nicotine Gum
	Zyban
Counseling	Group Counseling
	Individual Counseling
	Telephone Counseling

Tobacco and the Future of Business

Tobacco use is declining in the United States and in most industrialized countries. The intelligent businessperson will see this change as an opportunity and take advantage of the situation. Over 80 percent of consumers are nonsmokers; they, and most of the rest, oppose marketing and selling tobacco to children. Companies currently selling cigarettes could team up with other (nontobacco) companies to market new products. For example, the highly valuable shelf space behind the cashier of a convenience store could be used for iPod accessories, cell phone accessories, or the latest video games or DVDs, instead of for tobacco. A tobacco-free store would bring an entirely different clientele and would stand out from its competitors.

The Target Corporation stopped selling tobacco products in 1996. Since then, sales at Target increased from $474 million to $52 billion. Only the boldest and most daring retailers, convenience stores, grocery stores, drug stores, or service stations will take the leap and eliminate tobacco sales, but those stores that do so and that replace tobacco with products of the future will come out on top of their market in the end.

The Future of Enforcement

All states have some form of legislation outlawing tobacco sales to minors. However, in undercover purchases by the police, 10 to 30 percent of the time, or more, minors buy cigarettes. The United States Department of Health and Human Services Healthy People 2010 initiative set a goal to reduce this level to 5 percent or less. If a bar or liquor store made underage sales of alcohol over 10 percent of the time, they would very likely be closed down. Stores caught selling tobacco to children usually only get warnings or small fines.

Where a Tobacco Dollar Goes

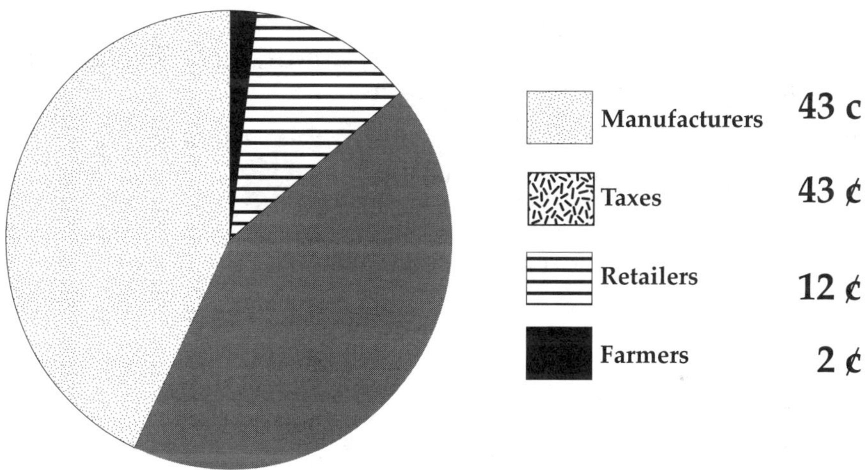

Figure 8.2 Chart showing where a tobacco dollar goes. From each dollar spent by the consumer, most of the money goes to the tobacco companies and to taxes and only 2 percent to the farmers.

Tobaccofreekids.org lists the following key steps to controlling underage sales:

- **Mandatory participation by all tobacco retailers.**
- **Designating an agency in the state with clear responsibility for enforcement.**
- **Providing adequate, guaranteed funding for enforcement**
- **Licensing of vendors by the enforcing agency; licensing should be self-supporting.**
- **Making frequent and realistic compliance checks, with a goal of 95 percent compliance.**
- **Meaningful penalties including graduated fines and ultimately, license suspension.**
- **No preemption of local ordinances.**
- **Education and awareness efforts for merchants and the public.**

Communities that have gotten serious about underage sales and followed these approaches have experienced dramatic decreases in tobacco use by children without harming local businesses. A research group from DePaul University found that a comprehensive youth access program in Woodridge, Illinois, reduced tobacco sales to minors from 70 percent to less than 5 percent in one-and-a-half years, and also reduced smoking among youth by over 50 percent.

The Future of Smoking in Public

As described in Chapter 6, smoking has been banned in the workplace, including bars and restaurants, in fourteen states, the District of Columbia, and Puerto Rico. Smoking has also been banned in many large cities like Chicago; Tucson; Honolulu; Lexington, Kentucky; Montgomery County, Maryland; Minneapolis; Bozeman; Albuquerque; and Austin. Smoke-free movements are springing up in nearly every state, and over the next several years smoking in the workplace will be outlawed in more and more states.

Several organizations concerned with cancer and health have begun holding their meetings and conferences exclusively in smoke-free states or cities. Beginning in 2007, the National Cancer Institute will require the meetings they sponsor to be held in smoke-free locations, joining the American Public Health Association, the Canadian Public Health Association, and the Office on Smoking and Health of the Centers for Disease Control and Prevention. This added economic pressure is likely to increase the pace in which states and cities enact smoking bans.

Many civic and fraternal organizations, such as the Elks, Eagles, and Masons, are experiencing a decline in members as the old members are not replaced by young people. Our local Elks Lodge sponsored the Boy Scout troop of my two sons. I learned of many very worthy activities that the Elks performed in our community. But the bar in the Elks Lodge is a ghastly, smoke-filled place that certainly had no appeal to me. Some lodges have banned smoking at their facilities and this has resulted in a resurgence in attendance and membership.

The Future of Tobacco Farming

The decline in tobacco use has important implications for farmers. Tobacco has been an important crop for certain regions of the country for hundreds of years. Of the 873 million pounds produced in the United States in 2003, 93 percent was grown in six states (North Carolina, Kentucky, Tennessee, Virginia, South Carolina, and Georgia). The total value of tobacco grown in the United States is $1.7 billion. However, for every dollar spent on cigarettes, only one cent goes to the farmer. Furthermore, 297 million pounds of tobacco are imported into the United States annually. The state of Maryland implemented a voluntary buyout program to switch tobacco farmers to other crops. Tobacco was the dominant crop in Southern Maryland and other forms of agriculture were underdeveloped. By paying farmers $1 per pound for ten years to stop growing tobacco (about half the average price), Maryland has gone from producing fifty-three million pounds in the 1950s to one million pounds in 2005. Farmers learned to grow other crops, and some have put in greenhouses to grow high-value plants, or have set up agritourism or equestrian businesses. Owners were also given incentives to put their land into an agriculture land conservation program, to maintain the land in farming.

New markets are developing for fresh vegetables, herbs, mushrooms, and spices. Tobacco was originally grown, in part, for its potential medicinal properties, and there are many other plants with medicinal value. It is interesting that several anticancer drugs are isolated from plants. Taxol is a drug isolated from the Pacific yew tree, a type of evergreen found on the Western coast of the United States. Taxol is effective in treating certain breast, lung, colon, and ovarian cancers. The corn lily plant, also found in the Western United States, produces a drug called cyclopamine, which is being developed to treat pancreas, stomach, and some prostate and lung tumors. It would be very exciting if farmers switched from growing tobacco to growing plants containing anticancer drugs!

There is also considerable interest in tobacco for biotechnology. Tobacco is one of the easiest plants to manipulate genetically, and several companies are using the tobacco plant to produce chemicals, pharmaceuticals, plastics, and new food ingredients. For this use, the tobacco plant is used as a biological factory to produce a compound which is then purified from the plant. This new field, molecular farming, is projected to grow into a $100 million business by the year 2020 (www.molecularfarming.com).

If a 1 percent tax was applied to all tobacco products and put into a fund to assist farmers in growing alternative crops and to educate them in alternative land uses, the transition could be accomplished more easily. A more diverse agriculture could be fostered, more land could be put into agricultural conservation, and more jobs for younger farmers would be generated.

The Future of the Tobacco Business

Last year, I was asked to give a presentation at a local Catholic school's career fair. I set up a table with some examples of my research on a childhood lung disease and some of the material on the effect of smoking on infants. Groups of five to ten middle school students came by my table and listened to my presentation and asked questions. I was struck by how many of them told me about relatives who smoke: their parents, aunts, uncles, and grandparents. It was unsettling to see these children receiving mixed messages. Their teachers and other adults are telling them about the dangers of smoking, yet they see adults in their home using tobacco.

However, the most surprising thing these students told me was in response to my asking them, "What should we as a society or community do to protect infants from the danger they are exposed to by tobacco use?" Two of the students came right out and said, "We should make tobacco illegal." I admit that I was caught off guard by this answer, but of course that is a perfectly logical response. For any other commercial product in our country, a clear danger to the user, when the product is used as intended, is sufficient cause to have the product severely regulated or outlawed. But I explained to the students that making tobacco illegal would undoubtedly fail, as people would smoke anyway. And a tobacco ban would lead to considerable illegal activity and crime, making the problem worse.

Many experts have pondered what the future of the tobacco industry will or should be. Dr. David Kessler, former head of the FDA, devotes the final chapter of his book, *A Question of Inte*nt to this topic. The book was written just after he left the FDA, and the battle to have cigarettes and nicotine regulated as a drug had failed. But the tobacco companies had just lost the first really large lawsuit, and many in the tobacco industry thought they might all go bankrupt.

Dr. Kessler came to the idea that the tobacco companies should be dismantled and a government-regulated cigarette production company be put in their place. Cigarettes would remain legal, be sold in plain wrappers with health warnings, and be sold strictly to adults.

No advertising or marketing of tobacco would be allowed, and the profits would all go into production, payment of legal judgments, medical research, and education. Dr. Kessler reasoned that as long as the companies had access to large amounts of money from tobacco profits, they would succeed in lobbying against restrictions and would market their products to young people.

Of course, the companies did not go bankrupt. They settled out of court with the states and now pump billions of dollars into state coffers. Big tobacco has been allowed to stay in business. The companies have changed their tune and admitted that nicotine is addictive and that cigarettes do cause cancer. But, they argue, as long as the product is legal and adults want to smoke, they will provide the customer what they want.

Gone is the Philip Morris that once boasted of 'having more money than God.' In its place is a multinational company increasingly buying tobacco, producing cigarettes and selling them internationally. As the United States market gradually shrinks, smokers in other countries have taken their place.

Like so many other public health issues, the best solutions lie not in government regulation and protection, but in our homes and communities. Parents need to explain to their children why they should not smoke, and lead by example. Parents must also protect their children from smoke and reduce their exposure to cigarette marketing. Magazines with tobacco ads will only exist if people buy them; stores will listen if consumers demand change and take their money elsewhere. Individual communities are changing laws and insisting that government enforce the laws we have.

Tobacco and smokers will surely be around for many years to come. As long as there are smokers, someone will grow the plant and someone will produce and sell the cigarettes. At the same time, tobacco does not have to be the number one cause of infant mortality and the number one cause of cancer, lung disease, and heart disease. That **can** change if we make it happen.

Title: Some of the young girls who roll cigarettes.

I could not induce the very smallest ones to get into the photo.
One boy said, "Lots are working under 14. I went in under 12."

Danville, Va., 06/06/1911

Photograph by Lewis Hine

Source-National Archives

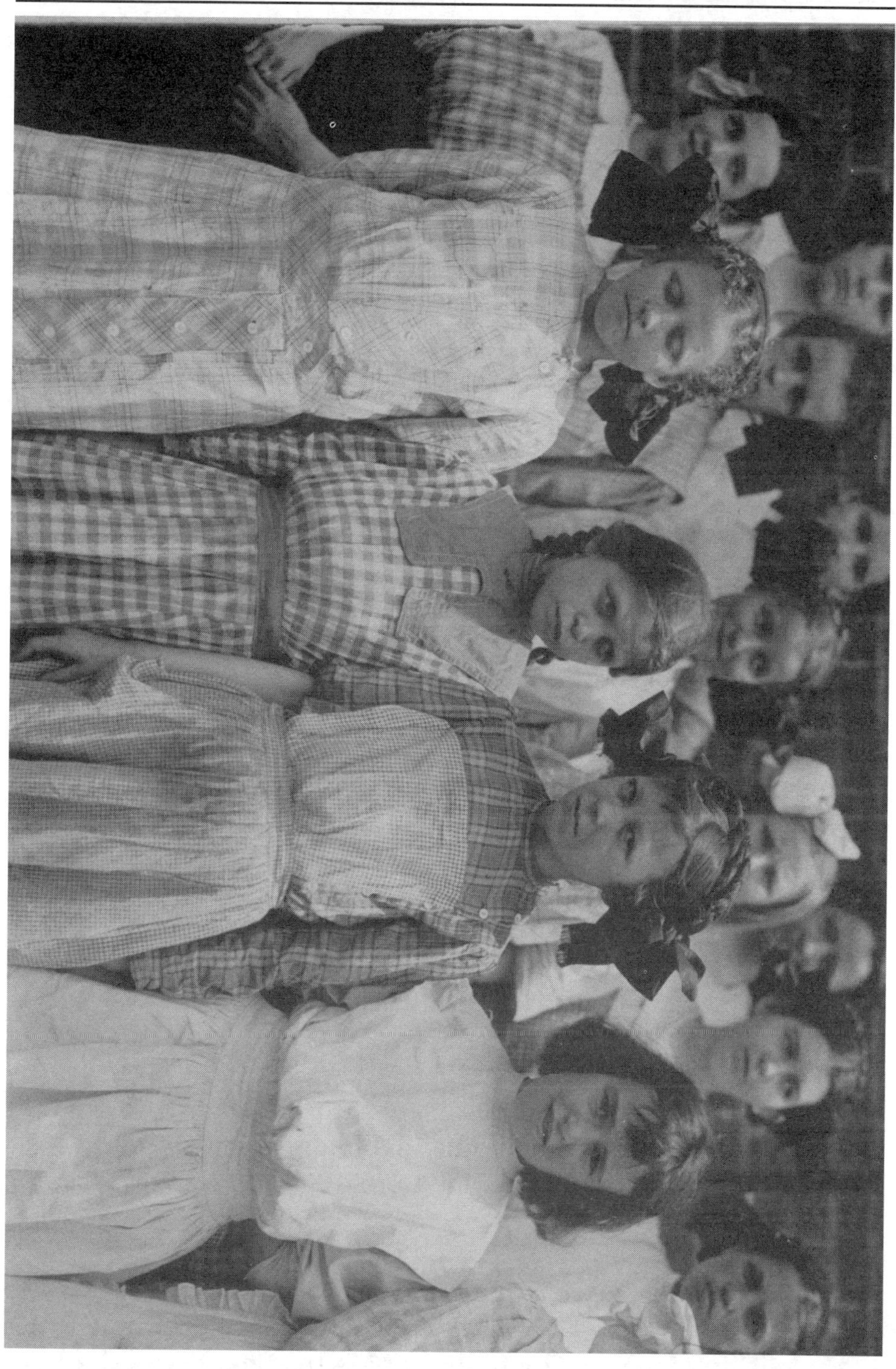

APPENDIX

I. Glossary

1-800-QUIT-NOW—Toll-free number connecting smokers to local quit smoking resources. The number works in all fifty states, Washington D.C., and Puerto Rico.

Abdominal aortic aneurysms—Ballooning of an artery, typically in the lower half of the body, often accompanied by back, stomach or groin pain. Occurs more frequently in men, especially if they have high blood pressure. If the artery ruptures, most patients will die before they get to the hospital.

Addiction—The repeated use of a substance or behavior despite harmful consequences. Some researchers apply 'addiction' only to the abuse of drugs and alcohol; others extend it to include behaviors such as overeating or gambling. Physically addicting substances produce a characteristic set of withdrawal symptoms when the user stops using the drug. Any pleasurable substance or activity can create a psychological addiction.

Adrenaline—A compound produced by the body's adrenal gland, also known as epinephrine. Secreted as part of a stress response stimulated by threats or excitement, it causes sweating, increases heart rate and raises blood sugar levels.

Age-related macular degeneration—A disorder leading to gradual vision loss. The most common cause of blindness in the elderly. Risk factors include smoking, high blood pressure, and a family history of the disease.

Bupropion—The generic name for Wellbutrin and Zyban. A drug originally developed as an anti-depressant but later found to be effective in smoking cessation. Bupropion treatment typically lasts for seven to twelve weeks, with the smoker stopping the use of tobacco around ten days into the treatment. The drug can be used in combination with nicotine replacement therapy and counseling.

Carbon monoxide—A colorless, odorless, tasteless, and highly toxic gas. It is a major product of the incomplete burning of substances such as tobacco, gasoline, or kerosene. Carbon monoxide causes poisoning by replacing oxygen in the major oxygen-containing protein in the blood, called hemoglobin. Carbon monoxide binds more tightly to hemoglobin than oxygen, so the poison can build up in the body, leading to oxygen starvation, damage to the heart, and — in high doses — brain damage and death. Most homes are now required to have a carbon monoxide detector to prevent poisoning.

Centers for Disease Control and Prevention (CDC)—A US Government agency in the Department of Health and Human Services, located in Atlanta, Georgia. The CDC is responsible for the identification and prevention of disease, especially infectious disease, and cooperates with the Surgeon General's office to produce the Surgeon General's Report on Smoking and Health.

Chronic obstructive pulmonary disease (COPD)—A group of lung diseases, including bronchitis and emphysema characterized by obstruction of the airways and reduced breathing capacity. The major cause of COPD is smoking and about 15 percent of smokers will develop the disease if they smoke long enough. It can also be caused by coal dust exposure.

Ectopic pregnancy—Development of a fertilized egg outside of the womb. The fetus typically implants in the fallopian tubes but can also implant in the cervix, abdomen, or ovaries. Smoking increases the risk of ectopic pregnancy.

Excise tax—A type of tax imposed on physical goods such as gasoline, alcohol, and tobacco. Often used as a way to discourage the use of harmful products ('sin tax'). The Federal tax on tobacco is $0.39 per pack, and city and state taxes vary by locality.

Fagerstrom Test for Nicotine Dependence—A seven-question test developed by Dr. Karl Fagerstrom to determine a person's level of nicotine addiction.

Fetal alcohol syndrome—Now known as fetal alcohol spectrum disorder. A group of birth defects caused by drinking alcohol during pregnancy. Drinking at any time during pregnancy can cause brain damage, as the baby's brain is developing throughout pregnancy. Features include facial deformities, delayed physical and emotional development, and memory and attention defects. Fetal alcohol exposure is the leading cause of mental retardation, and women are recommended to abstain from any alcohol consumption during pregnancy or if they plan to become pregnant.

The Food and Drug Administration (FDA)—A Government agency, part of the Department of Health and Human Services. The FDA regulates food, drugs, cosmetics, medical devices, and blood products.

Folic acid— An essential vitamin, that is particularly important for the developing brain of the fetus. Women need to take supplemental vitamins before and during pregnancy to ensure that they have adequate amounts.

Infant mortality— Death of a child in the first year of life.

James Buchanan "Buck" Duke (1856-1925) —North Carolina business man who licensed the first cigarette-rolling machine and built the American Tobacco Company. American Tobacco grew to have a virtual monopoly on the US cigarette market. In 1906, it was found guilty of antitrust violations, and the company was split up. In 1924, he donated the endowment forming Duke University.

Low birth weight—An infant born below the weight of 2500 grams (5.5 pounds). Smoking is the most common preventable cause of low birth weight.

Lung cancer—Any of several types of malignancy of the lung tissue. The most frequent cancer killer of both men and women, responsible for about 160 thousand deaths per year in the United States. Most lung cancer is caused by smoking. Asbestos exposure, radon, and certain occupational toxins have also been linked to lung cancer.

Lyme disease—A group of diseases caused by infection with a bacterium, Most often transmitted by the bite of a black-legged tick, also known as a deer tick. Initial symptoms often include a rash at the site of the bite; later symptoms include fever, and joint and muscle pain. Lyme disease can be transmitted from mother to fetus and can be fatal.

Meningococcal infections—Also known as bacterial meningitis. A bacterial infection from the organism *Neisseria meningitidis* that can be fatal or cause permanent disability. Smoking and secondhand smoke exposure are risk factors.

Miscarriage or spontaneous abortion—Death of the fetus in the uterus.

Molecular farming—The use of plants to produce new, non-food products, such as medicines or plant-based vaccines; to detect and remove soil toxins; and to produce chemicals. Tobacco plants are particularly well suited to molecular farming (see www.molecularfarming.com).

Neonatal period—The period from birth to twenty-eight days.

Neural tube defects—Any of a group of birth defects involving the development of the brain and nervous system. During development of the embryo a structure called the neural tube forms and gives rise to the brain and spinal cord. Defects in this process can lead to brain malformations or spina bifida. Neural tube defects are far less common in women taking regular doses of folic acid, a B vitamin. In the US, most grain products are enriched in folic acid, resulting in an estimated 25 percent reduction in neural tube defects.

Nicotine—The active drug in tobacco. Nicotine binds directly to specific receptors in the brain. The brain adapts to this stimulus, and addiction results. Withdrawal of nicotine causes the individual to feel a missing need. Nicotine responses differ among individuals, in part because of genetic differences in the breakdown of nicotine by the body.

Nicotine replacement therapy—A class of therapies to aid in quitting smoking. Nicotine is delivered in gum, patches, lozenges or nasal spray.

Placental abruption—A condition where the placenta tears away from the uterus. The condition occurs in about 1 percent of pregnancies worldwide and can lead to death of the fetus 20 to 40 percent of the time. Placental abruption can cause blood loss and other complications in the mother. Risk factors include high blood pressure, accidents, alcohol, and tobacco use. The condition is most common in mothers younger than twenty or older than thirty-five.

Placenta Previa—A pregnancy complication where the placenta blocks the cervix. A major cause of vaginal bleeding in the late stages of pregnancy. In severe cases, can lead to the need for emergency delivery of the baby. Smoking and cocaine use increase the risk.

Post neonatal period—The period starting twenty-eight days after birth and ending at twelve months of age.

The Pure Food and Drug Act—A federal law regulating meat products, food additives and drugs. Led to the creation of the Food and Drug Administration.

Relative risk of addiction—A scale of a drug's potential for addiction. The scale ranges from one, for low-risk drugs like caffeine, to five, for such highly addictive drugs such as cocaine.

Respiratory syncytial virus (RSV)—A common virus causing infant and childhood respiratory disease. In most children, infection leads to mild symptoms, but some cases can result in severe disease, hospitalization and, in some cases, death. Maternal smoking and exposure to tobacco smoke increase the risk of severe disease.

Sin taxes—Slang term for excise taxes targeted to reduce harmful behaviors such as alcohol or tobacco use or gambling.

Smoke Free Movies—A web site (www.smokefreemovies.ucsf.edu) featuring information on tobacco use in movies. The site proposes that movies with tobacco use be given an R rating.

Sudden infant death syndrome (SIDS)—The sudden death of an infant less than one year of age that remains unexplained after a medical examination.

Spina bifida—see Neural tube defects. A defect in the development of the spinal cord. Spina bifida can range in severity from mild nerve and muscle impairment to severe disabilities. The cause of spina bifida is unknown, but folic acid in the diet early in pregnancy can prevent the condition.

Taxol—The trade name for the drug paclitaxel, originally isolated from the Pacific Yew tree. Taxol is used to treat certain lung, ovarian and breast cancers. Taxol was originally discovered by the National Cancer Institute as part of a search for new cancer drugs naturally occurring in plants and other organisms.

Tobacco quota system—Following the Great Depression, price support and quotas were put in place for a number of crops, including tobacco. The quota system is being phased out, and a free market system will replace it.

Tobaccofreekids.org—Web site for the Campaign for Tobacco Free Kids, one of the largest private charities devoted to reducing tobacco addiction in children and to prevent secondhand smoke exposure.

We Card program—A voluntary program that many retail stores participate in, providing training for salespeople on avoiding the sale of tobacco products to underage buyers.

II. Statistics on Smoking and Infant Mortality

Proven associations of passive smoking affecting children*

Increased incidence of obstetric complications
Reduced birth weight
Reduced head circumference at birth
Increased incidence of SIDS
Increased incidence of meningococcal infections
Increased incidence of acute lower airway infections (birth to three years)
Increased incidence of middle ear disease
Increased incidence of wheezing (birth to five years)
More frequent respiratory symptoms (five to sixteen years)
Persisting reduced lung function

* Evidence obtained from well-designed cohort or case-control analytical studies, preferably from more than one center or research group. From the Surgeon General's Report on Smoking, 2001.

III. Surgeon General's List of Diseases Caused by Smoking

Proven associations between smoking and adult disease.

Cancer
Lung Cancer
Bladder cancer
Cervical cancer
Kidney cancer
Cancer of the larynx
Mouth and throat cancer
Acute Myeloid Leukemia
Pancreatic cancer
Stomach cancer

Cardiovascular disease
Abdominal aortic aneurysms
Atherosclerosis
Stroke
Coronary heart disease

Respiratory disease
Acute respiratory illness, including pneumonia
Impaired lung growth in childhood and adolescence
Lung function decline in late adolescence and early adulthood
Respiratory and asthma-related symptoms in children and adolescents including coughing and wheezing
Chronic obstructive pulmonary disease (COPD)

Reproductive effects
Sudden infant death syndrome
Fetal growth restriction and low birth weight
Reduced fertility in women
Premature rupture of membranes, placenta previa, and placental abruption
Preterm delivery and shortened gestation

Ophthalmologic (eye diseases)
Age-related macular degeneration and cataracts

General
Increased absenteeism and increased use of medical services
Risks of adverse surgical outcomes related to wound healing and respiratory complications
Hip fractures
Low bone density in postmenopausal women
Peptic ulcer disease in *Helicobacter pylori*-positive individuals

From United States Surgeon General's 2004 report on tobacco

http://www.cdc.gov/tobacco/sgr/sgr_2004/chapters.htm

IV. Healthy Mothers, Healthy Babies

Before Pregnancy

Get a prepregnancy checkup and dental exam

A health care provider can make sure that you have no medical problems that need treatment, ensure that your vaccines are up to date, discuss the importance of a healthy diet, and recommend an exercise program. You may need to be tested for sexually transmitted diseases and other infections. If you have a family history of genetic disease, it can be discussed at this time.

It is important to have dental work done before pregnancy and to make sure that your gums are healthy.

Develop a healthy diet, including a multivitamin with folic acid

A healthy diet and maintaining a healthy weight is very important in pregnancy. Avoid high-fat and high-sugar foods, cut back on caffeine and soda, and start drinking water regularly.

A multivitamin with 400 micrograms of folic acid taken once a day before pregnancy and during the first weeks of pregnancy can dramatically reduce the risk of several birth defects such as scoliosis and neural tube defects. Foods such as orange juice, fortified cereals, green vegetables, and beans also add folic acid to the diet (http://www.marchofdimes.com/pnhec/173_769.asp).

Choosing a multivitamin—(from the March of Dimes web site) http://www.marchofdimes.com/pnhec/173_15354.asp.

Start a regular exercise program

Beginning a regular exercise program before pregnancy can help you attain or maintain a healthy weight, and help you remain healthy during the pregnancy.

Stop smoking

Smoking and exposure to secondhand smoke reduce your fertility and harm the fetus and the baby. It is very important to stop smoking before pregnancy.

Stop drinking

Alcohol can also cause developmental problems in the baby, so it is best to stop drinking before pregnancy.

Stop taking illegal drugs

Many illegal drugs harm the baby and reduce fertility.

Avoid Infections

Wash your hands frequently.

Wash fruits and vegetables, and avoid raw or undercooked meats, fish and seafood.

Avoid handling cat litter or soil where cats go (sandboxes).

Avoid children with colds and infections.

Protect yourself from sexually transmitted diseases.

Avoid tick bites, as they can transmit Lyme disease and other infections. See your doctor if you are bitten by a tick or develop an unexplained rash.

Reduce stress

Develop strategies to reduce stress before pregnancy, including relaxation, meditation, exercise, and prayer.

Avoid hazardous chemicals

Some cleaning products, paints, and drinking water with lead can harm the baby.

Discuss any of these potential situations with a health care provider.

After you are Pregnant

Medical Care

Attend your regular prenatal care appointments. Regular check-ups can help answer questions, monitor important health parameters (blood pressure, blood sugar, weight gain), monitor the health of the baby, and provide referrals to health services.

Typical pregnancies will involve one doctor's visit each month for the first seven months and then one every week or two until the baby is born.

Inform your health care provider about any prescription or over-the-counter medications you are taking. Many medications are not safe to take during pregnancy.

Diet and Exercise

Most women need about 300 extra calories per day while pregnant. A healthy diet is important to ensure proper growth of the baby. An example of such a diet is shown here: (http://www.marchofdimes.com/pnhec/159_823.asp).

Certain foods that are high in toxins or that might contain infectious agents are not recommended. These include fish that might be high in mercury, such as swordfish, shark, king mackerel, and local game fish such as trout, salmon, and bass. Raw fish, particularly oysters and clams should not be eaten, nor should undercooked meats or deli meats that have not been cooked, soft cooked eggs, or foods with raw eggs. Soft cheeses such as Brie or feta, should be avoided, along with unpasteurized milk, juices, or raw sprouts. Herbal supplements and teas should also be avoided.

Take the daily prenatal vitamins given to you by your health care provider. In addition you may be given a calcium supplement.

Most women can continue their regular exercise program during most of the pregnancy. Walking, swimming, biking, aerobics, and yoga are good choices. Avoid sports with a high risk of injury. Follow the advice of your health care provider. Exercise can reduce the risk of gestational diabetes and stress. If you experience vaginal bleeding, dizziness, headaches, chest pain, decreased fetal movement, or contractions, seek immediate medical care.

Drink no more than two cups of coffee, tea, or caffeine containing soda per day. Water, milk, and juices are better choices. Avoid over-the-counter medications containing caffeine.

Alcohol

Drinking during pregnancy can cause fetal alcohol syndrome resulting in physical abnormalities and learning disabilities. This is a leading cause of mental retardation.

There is no known safe level of alcohol exposure, so experts recommend that women who are pregnant or trying to become pregnant refrain from drinking all alcoholic beverages. For the Surgeon General's report on the topic see http://www.hhs.gov/surgeongeneral/pressreleases/sg02222005.html

Herbs and preparations

Many herbs, including herbal teas, are not safe to take during pregnancy.

V. Magazines Without Tobacco Advertising

Ability Magazine
Adbusters
Air and Space
Alaska Magazine
American Baby
Alternative Medicine Digest
American Art Review
American Cowboy Magazine
The American Gardener
American History Illustrated
Archaeology
Arthritis Today
Arthur Frommer's Budget Travel
Audubon
Aviation Week and Space Technology
B&W Magazine
Baby Talk
Backpacker
Better Homes and Gardens
Bicycling
Biography
Birders' World
Bonkers
Boy's Life
Canoe & Kayak magazine
Cat Fancy
Catholic Digest
Cats USA
Classic American Homes
Consumer Reports
Consumer Reports on Health
Crafts
Custom Home
Cyclist
Dawn East Magazine
Decorator Showcase
Diabetes
Diabetes Forecast
Diet and Exercise
Discover
Dog Fancy
Downbeat
Early American Life
The Economist
Endless Vacation Magazine
Entrepreneur
Everyday Food
Exercise for Men Only
Extra!
FDA Consumer
Family Fun
Family PC
Farm Journal
Film Comment
Fine Cooking
Fine Gardening
Fishing Facts
Fit
Fit Pregnancy
Fitness
Focus on Healthy Aging
Food and Fitness Advisor

The Futurist
Golf Digest
Golf Illustrated
Golf Week
Golf World
The Grapevine Magazine
Grace Woman
Guide Posts
Guitar Player
Hadassah Magazine
Harvard Business Review
Harvard Medical School Health Letter
Health
Health Letter
Healthy Weight Journal
Healthy & Natural Journal
Healthy Kids
Healthy Pregnancy
The Herb Companion
Highlights for Children
The Hightower Lowdown
The Historian
Historic Preservation
Hit Parader
Home Magazine
Home Office Computing
House Beautiful
Horticulture
Humpty Dumpty's Magazine
International Travel News
Isaac Asimov's Science Fiction
Jack and Jill
Kiplinger's Personal Finance
Living Fit
Magazine of Fantasy and Science Fiction
Maximum Golf
Mayo Clinic Health Letter
Medical Economics
Medical Self-care
Men's Fitness
Men's Health
Men's Health Advisor
Men's Journal
Metropolitan Home
Model Railroader
Modern Maturity
Money
Mother Earth News
Mother Jones
Mothering
Motor Boating
Mountain Bike
Ms.
Museum
Mutual Funds
The Nation
National Geographic
National Geographic Adventure
National Geographic Traveler
National Journal
National Parks Journal
National Wildlife
Nation's Business
Natural Health
Natural History
Natural Living Today

Nature
Nature Conservancy
New Age
New Scientist
Nick Jr.
North American Review
Nutrition Action Healthletter
Oceans
Old House Journal
ONE Magazine
Organic Style
Outside
Oxygen Magazine
PC Magazine
PC World
Parent And Child
Personal Computing
Popular Communications
Popular Photography
Preservation
Prevention
Priorities for Health
Psychology Today
Railfan and Railroad
Ranger Rick
Real Sports
Regional Review
Runner's World
Sail
Saturday Evening Post
Science
Science News
The Sciences
Scientific American
The Scientific Review of Alternative Medicine
Sea Kayaker Magazine
Sierra
Ski Magazine
Skiing Magazine
Smart Computing
Smart Money
Smithsonian
Sound And Vision
STOP! 'The New Magazine for Smokers Who Want to Stop'
Stork
Sunset Magazine
T&L Golf (Travel + Leisure Magazine)
Theater Crafts
Thrasher Skateboard Magazine
Threads
Today's Health and Wellness Magazine
Town and Country
Traditional Home
Tufts University Health & Nutrition Letter
Trains
Travel
Travel and Leisure
Trust
Trusts and Estates
Twist
Vegetarian Resource Journal
Vegetarian Times

Victoria
The Washingtonian Magazine
The Washington Monthly
Weight Watchers
Western Outdoors
Women's Fitness International
Women's Health Advisor
The World Today
Worst Pills, Best Pills News
Writer's Digest
YM (Young and Modern)
Yachting Magazine
Yankee
Your Health

VI. Organizations Involved in Anti-Tobacco and Smoking Cessation

Action on Smoking and Health
http://ash.org

The Advocacy Institute
http://www.advocacy.org/publications/mtc

American Cancer Society
http://www.cancer.org

American Council on Science and Health
http://www.acsh.org/healthissues

The American Heart Association
http://www.americanheart.org

The American Legacy Foundation
http://www.americanlegacy.org
http://www.thetruth.com

The American Lung Association
http://www.lungusa.org

Americans for Nonsmokers' Rights
http://www.no-smoke.org Has a page with grades on each state for tobacco control laws (http://lungaction.org/reports/tobacco-control04.html)

The Campaign for Tobacco Free Kids
http://tobaccofreekids.org

The Centers for Disease Control and Prevention – Office on Smoking and Health (OSH)
http://www.cdc.gov/tobacco

The Center for Tobacco Control Research and Education
http://repositories.cdlib.org

The Foundation for a Smokefree America
http://www.tobaccofree.org
http://www.notobacco.org

get outraged
Site for teens sponsored by the Massachusetts Department of Public Health
http://www.getoutraged.com/

International Union Against Cancer
http://www.globalink.org

The Legacy Tobacco Documents Library
http://legacy.library.ucsf.edu

The National Association of African Americans for Positive Imagery (NAAAPI)
http://www.naaapi.org/tobacco

The National Latino Council on Alcohol and Tobacco Prevention (LCAT)
http://www.nlcatp.org

The Partnership for a Drug Free America
http://www.drugfree.org/Intervention/Drug_Guide/Tobacco

The PATCH Project — Program Against Teen Chewing
http://homepage.mac.com/craigstotts/patchproject

National Cancer Institute
http://www.cancer.gov

Robert Wood Johnson Foundation/Smoke-free Families
http://www.rwjf.org
http://www.smokefreefamilies.org

Smokefree.net
http://www.smokefree.net

Tobacco Free Nurses
http://tobaccofreenurses.org

The Tobacco Technical Assistance Consortium (TTAC)
http://www.ttac.org

The United States Surgeon General
http://www.surgeongeneral.gov/tobacco/

The Virginia Tobacco Settlement Foundation
http://www.vtsf.org

The World Health Organization (WHO)
http://www.who.int/tobacco

YdoYouThink

Site for kids sponsored by The Virginia Tobacco Settlement Foundation
http://www.whydoyouthink.com

VII. Child Health and SIDS Support Groups

The American SIDS Institute
http://www.sids.org

The Association of Maternal and Child Health Programs
http://www.amchp.org

The Committee on Native American Child Health (CONACH)
http://www.aap.org/nach

KidsHealth
http://www.kidshealth.org

March of Dimes
http://www.marchofdimes.com

The National Center for Education in Maternal and Child Health
http://www.ncemch.org

The National Institute of Child Health and Human Development (NICHD)
http://www.nichd.nih.gov

The National SIDS & Infant Death Project IMPACT
http://www.sidsprojectimpact.com

SIDS Network
http://sids-network.org

WIC— Women, Infants, and Children
http://www.fns.usda.gov/wic

VIII. Lung Disease and Lung Cancer Foundations and Resources

The Asbestos Disease Awareness Organization
http://www.mesolung.org

The Belanger-Federico-Pitterich Foundation
http://www.belangerfederico.org

Emphysema and COPD (Chronic Obstructive Pulmonary Disease)
http://health.nih.gov/result.asp

Lung Cancer Alliance
http://www.lungcanceralliance.org

Lung Cancer Online Foundation
http://www.lungcanceronline.org

The LUNGevity Foundation
http://www.lungevity.org

National Cancer Institute
http://www.cancer.gov/cancertopics/types/lung

VIII. Smoking Cessation Resources

Smokefree.gov
http://www.smokefree.gov
The US Government's central online guide to quitting

The American Legacy Foundation
http://www.americanlegacy.org/
Non-profit foundation started from tobacco settlement funds with programs for youth and adults wishing to quit.

National Heart and Lung Institute
http://www.nhlbi.nih.gov/health/public/heart/other/chdblack/refresh.pdf
Quit-smoking guide

Centers for Disease Control (CDC)
http://www.cdc.gov/tobacco/how2quit.htm
Central site at the CDC for smoking cessation resources.

Surgeon General
http://www.surgeongeneral.gov/tobacco/
The US Surgeon General's site for quit-smoking resources for the public and health care professionals. The site also has links to the Surgeon General's reports on smoking.

Nicotine Anonymous
http://www.nicotine-anonymous.org/
Nicotine Anonymous is a non-profit 12 step fellowship of men and women helping each other live nicotine-free lives.

Quitnet.com
http://www.quitnet.com/

An online community of smokers and ex-smokers providing quit-smoking support, stop-smoking aids and expert advice.

Circle of Friends
http://www.join-the-circle.org
A program led by the American Legacy Foundation offering support for women smokers wanting to quit.

American Cancer Society
http://www.cancer.org
Extensive site from the American Cancer Society on reasons to quit, methods for quitting, and resources.

Center for Tobacco Cessation
http://www.ctcinfo.org
The American Cancer Society and the Robert Wood Johnson Foundation jointly fund the Center for Tobacco Cessation. The center serves as a source of science on tobacco cessation and works with national partners to expand the use of effective tobacco dependence treatments.

GottaQuit
http://www.gottaquit.com
Site for teens sponsored by the Monroe County, NY, Department of Health and the University of Rochester Medical Center.

Quit4Life
http://www.quit4life.com
Health Canada site for teen quitters. In both English and French

WhyQuit
http://whyquit.com
Site featuring information and resources for smokers to quit 'cold turkey."

Smoking cessation for pregnant women

National Partnership to Help Pregnant Smokers Quit
http://www.helppregnantsmokersquit.org
A group of organizations joined together to increase the number of pregnant smokers who quit.

Save Our Daughters
http://www.saveourdaughters.org
Sponsored by The Campaign for Tobacco-Free Kids, provides information on women and smoking and on reducing the impact of tobacco on women and girls.

Great Start
http://www.americanlegacy.org
Site from the American Legacy Foundation providing a program for pregnant women to stop smoking.

Smoke Free Families
http://www.smokefreefamilies.org
Smoke-Free Families is a national program supported by The Robert Wood Johnson Foundation working to discover the best ways to help pregnant smokers quit, and spread the word about effective, evidence-based treatments.

Sites for specific groups

Smoking Cessation, Quality of Life and Older Persons
http://www.tcsg.org/tobacco/cessation.htm
This site is intended to provide information on smoking cessation, the effects of smoking cessation on the health of older persons, and the value of healthy lifestyles for older persons, which include not smoking or being exposed to secondhand smoke.

Tobacco Free Nurses
http://www.tobaccofreenurses.org
Tobacco Free Nurses is the first national program focused on helping nurses and student nurses to stop smoking.

ChewFree.com
http://www.chewfree.com
A research project funded by the National Cancer Institute and the Oregon Research Institute to help people quit their use of chewing tobacco or snuff.

Commercial sites and products

Allen Carr's Easyway To Stop Smoking
http://www.theeasywaytostopsmoking.com
Information on Allen Carr smoking cessation seminars and a link to purchase the book.

Habitrol Nicotine patch-Novartis
http://www.habitrol.com
Information about the Habitrol nicotine patch as well as the Smokefree Program to help smokers quit.

NicoDerm CQ, GlaxoSmithKline Inc.
http://quit.com
GlaxoSmithKline site to promote Nicoderm (patch), Nicorette (gum), and Commit (lozenge) nicotine replacement therapy. Also contains smoking cessation information and resources.

Nicotrol-Nicotine nasal spray and inhaler, Pfizer, Inc.
http://www.nicotrol.com
Information on nicotine sprays and inhalers

Chantix, Pfizer, Inc.
http://www.chantix.com
Site for the smoking cessation drug Chantix. Contains a free smoking cessation counseling program designed for Chantix users.

Zyban-GlaxoSmithKline, Inc.
http://us.gsk.com
Site for the antidepressant drug Zyban used for smoking cessation.

Stop Smoking Today
http://www.stopsmokingtoday.com
Site featuring quitting information and links to purchase smoking cessation products.

QuitKey
http://www.quitkey.com/index.html
Site to purchase the QuitKey, a handheld device for recording smoking and to assist smokers in quitting.

IX. Mutual Funds and their Involvement in Tobacco

Tobacco Holdings and Grade for the 25 largest Mutual Funds

Size	Symbol	Fund	Altria %	Other Tobacco %	Grade
8	FMAGX	Fidelity Magellan	0	0	A
19	FDGRX	Fidelity Growth Company	0	0	A
25	FKINX	Franklin Income A	0	0	A
23	DODBX	Dodge & Cox Balanced	0	1.49	B
13	FLPSX	Fidelity Low-Priced Stock	0	1.63	B
4	FCNTX	Fidelity Contrafund	0	2.07	B
24	FPURX	Fidelity Puritan	0	2.26	B
22	FEQIX	Fidelity Equity-Income	0	3.38	B
17	FGRIX	Fidelity Growth & Income	0	3.54	B
6	DODGX	Dodge & Cox Stock	0	4.96	C
5	AWSHX	American Funds Washington Mutual A	0	5.58	C
16	VTSMX	Vanguard Total Stock Mkt Idx	1.08	2.46	D
7	AMECX	American Funds Inc Fund of Amer A	1.17	2.64	D
20	VWELX	Vanguard Wellington	1.23	2.48	D

Size	Symbol	Fund	Altria %	Other Tobacco %	Grade
10	CWGIX	American Funds Capital World G/I A	1.38	1.14	D
11	VINIX	Vanguard Institutional Index	1.38	3.09	D
2	VFINX	Vanguard 500 Index	1.38	3.1	D
12	VFIAX	Vanguard 500 Index Adm	1.38	3.1	D
1	AGTHX	American Funds Grth Fund of Amer A	1.43	0	D
15	ABALX	American Funds American Balanced A	1.51	6.02	F
9	CAIBX	American Funds Capital Inc Bldr A	1.56	0	F
14	ANWPX	American Funds New Perspective A	1.76	0	F
21	ANCFX	American Funds Fundamental Invs A	1.96	1.3	F
18	VWNFX	Vanguard Windsor II	2.51	5.11	F
3	AIVSX	American Funds Invmt Co of Amer A	4.71	1.44	F

Information from July 2006 obtained from Yahoo finance http://finance.yahoo.com/funds.

The twenty-five largest mutual funds by dollar value of holdings were identified from Yahoo Finance (a few bond-only funds and foreign funds were excluded). The top ten holdings of each fund were extracted and holdings of major tobacco companies were noted. Only Philip Morris/Altria-MO was found. Holdings in other companies making part of their income in the advertising, distribution, or marketing of tobacco were also identified. These companies include Berkshire Hathaway (BKS), Chevron (CVX), ConocoPhilips (COP), Exxon Mobil (XOM), Occidental Petroleum (OXY), and Royal Dutch Shell (RDS), Safeway (SWY), Time Warner (TWX), Wal-Mart (WMT). A grade of A was given to funds with no tobacco holdings, B to funds with less than 4 percent "Other tobacco," C to funds with more than 4 percent "Other tobacco," D to funds with 1 to 1.5 percent Altria, and F to funds with more than 1.5 percent Altria.

X. States and territories that have banned smoking in offices, bars, and restaurants

California
Colorado
Connecticut
Delaware
Hawaii
Maine
Massachusetts
Montana
New Jersey
New York
Puerto Rico
Rhode Island
Vermont
Utah
Washington
Washington D.C.

Arkansas, Florida, Georgia, Idaho, North Dakota, and Louisiana have smoke-free offices and restaurants; and South Dakota and Maryland, smoke-free offices.

XI. Countries with Smoking Bans

Bermuda
Bhutan
England
Ireland
Italy
Malta
New Zealand
Norway
Scotland
Spain
Sweden
Uganda
Uruguay
Wales

XII. Infant Mortality Statistics

Country	Rank	Deaths/1,000 births
Singapore	1	2.3
Sweden	2	2.8
Japan	4	3.2
Germany	11	4.1
Canada	23	4.7
Nonsmoking White Americans	**31**	**5.3**
United States (All)	43	6.4
Poland	52	7.2
Puerto Rico	66	9.4
White American Smokers	**72**	**9.8**
Ukraine	74	9.9
Native American Smokers	**78**	**12.1**
Russia	94	15.1
Jamaica	98	16.0
African American Smokers	**113**	**20.0**
Mexico	114	20.3
China	124	23.1
N. Korea	125	23.3
Libya	126	23.7

Data for US smokers and nonsmokers are from the CDC linked birth and death records for 2002. Other data are from the CIA World Fact Book for 2006 (www.cia.gov/cia/publications/factbook/rankorder/2091rank.html).

XIII. State Data on Taxes, Smoking Rates, and the Impact of Smoking

The CDC's Office on Smoking and Health maintains a web site supporting the efforts in each state to fund and carry out tobacco control policies called Sustaining State Funding for Tobacco Control. Within this site are data tables with information each state, last updated in the year 2004.

http://www.cdc.gov/tobacco/sustainingstates/FactsFinal.pdf

Data on smoking prevalence for adults and children in each state. Also shows the percentage of adults trying to quit, smoking-attributable deaths, youth projected to start smoking and projected to die from smoking.

http://www.cdc.gov/tobacco/datahighlights/page4.htm

Data on the percentage of residents in each state that smoke — by ethnicity, education level, income and age group.

http://www.cdc.gov/tobacco/datahighlights/page5.htm

Data on the cost of a pack of cigarettes in each state, workplace smoking policies, medical and productivity costs, and Medicaid costs.

http://www.cdc.gov/tobacco/datahighlights/Page6.htm

The National Conference of State Legislatures site, showing tobacco excise taxes across the nation.

http://www.ncsl.org/programs/health/cigarette.htm

State funding of tobacco prevention. The Campaign for Tobacco-Free Kids presents an annual report on the amount each state spends on tobacco prevention, the percentage of tax revenues spent, and trends over time.

http://www.tobaccofreekids.org/reports/settlements

XIV. Tobacco Company Subsidiaries and their Products

Altria/Philip Morris

Owns Kraft foods

Products sold by Kraft Foods (From their 2004 SEC filing)

Snacks: Oreo, Chips Ahoy!, Newtons, Peak Freans, Nilla, Nutter Butter, Stella D'Oro and SnackWell's cookies; Ritz, Premium, Triscuit, Wheat Thins, Cheese Nips, Better Cheddars, Honey Maid Grahams and Teddy Grahams crackers, Planters nuts, Terry's and Toblerone chocolates, Handi-Snacks, Fruit Snacks, and Balance Bar snacks.

Beverages: Maxwell House, General Foods International Coffees, Starbucks (under license), Yuban, Seattle's Best (under license), Sanka, Nabob and Gevalia coffees, Capri Sun (under license), Tang, Kool-Aid Crystal Light and Country Time juices and powdered beverages, Veryfine juices, Tazo teas (under license), and Fruit 2O water.

Cheese: Kraft and Cracker Barrel cheeses, Philadelphia cream cheese, Kraft and Velveeta processed cheeses, Kraft grated cheeses, Cheez Whiz, and Knudsen and Breakstone's cottage cheese and sour cream.

Grocery: Cool Whip; Back to Nature; Post cereals; Cream of Wheat and Cream of Rice; Kraft peanut butter; Miracle Whip, Kraft salad dressings; A.1. steak sauce; Kraft and Bull's-Eye barbecue sauces; Grey Poupon mustards; Shake 'N Bake; Jell-O desserts and pudding; Handi-Snacks and Milk-Bone pet snacks.

Loews Corporation/Carolina Group

Owns Loews hotels, CNA insurance, and Bulova watches

US Smokeless Tobacco

Owns International Wine and Spirits

Reference Books

Carr, Allen, *The Easy Way to Stop Smoking*: Join the Millions Who Have Become Nonsmokers Using the Easyway Method. Sterling Press, 2005.

Gately, Iain, *Tobacco: A Cultural History Of How An Exotic Plant Seduced Civilization*. Grove Press, New York 2001.

Glantz, Stanton A, John Slade, Lisa A. Bero, Peter Hanauer, Deborah E. Barnes, *The Cigarette Papers*. University of California Press, Berkeley 1988.

Kessler, David A., *A Question of Intent: A Great American Battle With a Deadly Industry*. Public Affairs, New York 2002.

Kluger, Richard, *Ashes to Ashes: America's Hundred-Year Cigarette War, the Public Health, and the Unabashed Triumph of Philip Morris*. Vintage Books, New York 1997.

Orey, Michael, *Assuming the Risk: The Mavericks, the Lawyers, and the Whistle-Blowers Who Beat Big Tobacco*. Little, Brown, Boston 1999.

Sullum, Jacob, *For Your Own Good; The Anti-smoking crusade and the tyranny of public health*. The Free Press, New York 1998.

Vanderhoof-Forschner, Karen, *Everything You Need to Know About Lyme Disease and Other Tick-Borne Disorders*. Wiley and Sons, Hoboken 2003.

Index

Symbols

A

B

C

D

E

F

G

H

Q

R

S

T

U

V

W

Z

About The Author

The author has a Bachelor of Arts degree from Boston University and a Ph.D. in Biochemistry from Boston University School of Medicine. Dr. Dean has been employed in the field of cancer research and human genetics in Frederick, Maryland for over 20 years.

Dr. Dean is an author on over 200 research articles in scientific journals and over 30 review articles and chapters in journals and books. He is a regular invited speaker at national and international scientific meetings and teaches at Hood College, the Johns Hopkins School of Medicine, and others. Dr. Dean is the author of an online book, *The Human ATP-binding Cassette Transporter Genes,* at the National Center for Biotechnology Information (www.ncbi.nlm.nih.gov/books). He is the recipient of the Young Investigator award from the American Association for Cancer Research and the National Institute of Health Director's Award. He holds five patents for the discovery of human disease genes. Dr. Dean is the founder of the NCI-Frederick's Elementary Outreach Program which has brought hands-on science lessons to over 10,000 students in Frederick County schools.

Dr. Dean's research team studies the genetic basis of human disease and has been involved in the cloning of the genes for cystic fibrosis, an inherited form of skin cancer, genes that cause kidney cancer, retinal degeneration, anemia, and genes involved in the resistance to Human Immunodeficiency Virus (HIV) and the progression to AIDS.

Dr. Dean is also an artist specializing in oil on canvas Pop Art paintings utilizing health, education, science, and environmental topics.

The Last Word and Acknowledgements

This book has been self-published. Why? Well no agent or publisher I contacted wanted to take it on. Besides, new authors have to do all the work to promote their books anyway.

I am a scientist, and this book is an experiment. Is there a message here people need to hear? Will people like the book and tell their friends? Will the media pick up some of these themes? Can I promote this thing, in my 'spare time,' without driving my family nuts? Stay tuned!

The book is part of a larger project, The Arts & Sciences Project, involving paintings and science museum-style exhibits. Maybe you can help bring The Project to our local art museum, science museum or university. All proceeds will go to promoting the project.

I did have several professionals help with this book. Midpoint Trade Books is the distributor (http://www.midpointtrade.com) and Gail Kump provided needed advice. The cover was designed by Janice Benight and Don Scott edited the manuscript.

A book produced by a major publisher goes through many rounds of copy editing, fact checking, and proof reading. That didn't happen with *Empty Cribs*, and any mistakes are my own. Feel free to send in corrections and together we'll make the next version better! The web site (www.artsciencepub.com) will have updates, corrections, and information on sources.

Lastly, I thank my parents for giving me a love of science and exploration. My children, Stephen, Jeff, and Laura are the inspiration for this book. And I thank my wife, Charlene, for her love, support, and seemingly endless tolerance (and editing).

—Frederick, MD 9/15/2006

Order Form

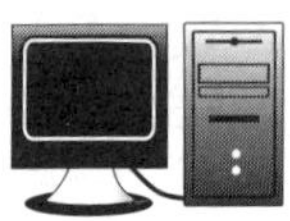

Email orders:

orders@artsciencepub.com

Mail orders:
Arts and Sciences Publishing
5257 Buckeystown Pike, Ste.173
Frederick, MD 21704

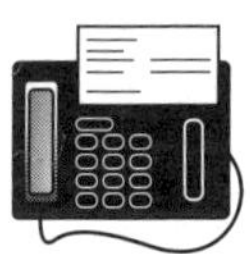

FAX orders:
1-301-620-8821

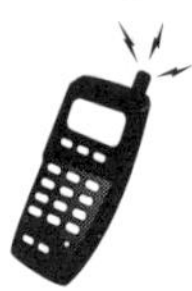

Phone orders

1-800-445-9832

Please send the following books. I understand I can return any of them for a full refund.

Empty Cribs	**1 book**	**$11.95**
	2-4 books	**$ 9.55 each**
	Larger quantities	**inquire**

Name:______________________________________

Address:____________________________________

City:_________________**State:**_________ **Zip:**_______

Telephone:___________________________________

Email:______________________________________

Sales Tax: Please add 5% for shipments to Maryland address. Shipping by air-U.S. $4.00 for first book, $2.00 for each additional book. International $6.00 for first book, $4.00 for each additional book.